Hypertrophic Cardiomyopathy

Editors

SRIHARI S. NAIDU
JULIO A. PANZA

CARDIOLOGY CLINICS

www.cardiology.theclinics.com

February 2019 • Volume 37 • Number 1

ELSEVIER

1600 John F. Kennedy Boulevard • Suite 1800 • Philadelphia, Pennsylvania, 19103-2899

http://www.theclinics.com

CARDIOLOGY CLINICS Volume 37, Number 1
February 2019 ISSN 0733-8651, ISBN-13: 978-0-323-65447-0

Editor: Stacy Eastman
Developmental Editor: Sara Watkins

Cardiology Clinics (ISSN 0733-8651) is published quarterly by Elsevier Inc., 360 Park Avenue South, New York, NY 10010-1710. Months of issue are February, May, August, and November. Business and Editorial Offices: 1600 John F. Kennedy Blvd., Ste. 1800, Philadelphia, PA 19103-2899. Customer Service Office: 3251 Riverport Lane, Maryland Heights, MO 63043. Periodicals postage paid at New York, NY and additional mailing offices. Subscription prices are $349.00 per year for US individuals, $672.00 per year for US institutions, $100.00 per year for US students and residents, $432.00 per year for Canadian individuals, $843.00 per year for Canadian institutions, $466.00 per year for international individuals, $843.00 per year for international institutions and $220.00 per year for Canadian and international students/residents. To receive student/resident rate, orders must be accompanied by name of affiliated institution, data of term, and the *signature* of program/residency coordinator on institution letterhead. Orders will be billed at individual rate until proof of status is received. Foreign air speed delivery is included in all *Clinics* subscription prices. All prices are subject to change without notice. **POSTMASTER:** Send address changes to *Cardiology Clinics*, Elsevier Health Sciences Division, Subscription Customer Service, 3251 Riverport Lane, Maryland Heights, MO 63043. **Customer Service: 1-800-654-2452 (U.S. and Canada); 314-447-8871 (outside U.S. and Canada). Fax: 314-447-8029. E-mail: journalscustomerservice-usa@ elsevier.com (for print support); journalsonlinesupport-usa@elsevier.com (for online support).**

Reprints. For copies of 100 or more, of articles in this publication, please contact the Commercial Reprints Department, Elsevier Inc., 360 Park Avenue South, New York, NY 10010-1710. Tel.: 212-633-3874; Fax: 212-633-3820; E-mail: reprints@elsevier.com.

Cardiology Clinics is also published in Spanish by McGraw-Hill Interamericana Editores S. A., P.O. Box 5-237, 06500, Mexico D. F., Mexico; in Portuguese by Reichmann and Alfonso Editores Rio de Janeiro, Brazil; and in Greek by Dimitrios P. Lagos, 8 Pondon Street, GR115-28 Ilissia, Greece.

Cardiology Clinics is covered in *MEDLINE/PubMed (Index Medicus), Excerpta Medica, The Cumulative Index to Nursing and Allied Health Literature* (CINAHL).

Contributors

EDITORIAL BOARD

JORDAN M. PRUTKIN, MD, MHS, FHRS
Assistant Professor of Medicine, Division of
Cardiology/Electrophysiology, UW Medical
Center, Seattle, Washington, USA

DAVID M. SHAVELLE, MD, FACC, FSCAI
Associate Professor, Keck School of Medicine
of USC, Director, General Cardiovascular
Fellowship Program, Director, Cardiac
Catheterization Laboratory, LAC + USC
Medical Center, Division of Cardiovascular
Medicine, University of Southern California,
Los Angeles, California, USA

TERRENCE D. WELCH, MD, FACC
Assistant Professor, Department of Medicine,
Section of Cardiology, Dartmouth-Hitchcock
Medical Center, Lebanon, New Hampshire,
USA; Department of Internal Medicine,
Dartmouth Geisel School of Medicine,
Hanover, New Hampshire, USA

AUDREY H. WU, MD
Assistant Professor, Internal Medicine,
University of Michigan, Ann Arbor, Michigan,
USA

EDITORS

SRIHARI S. NAIDU, MD, FACC, FAHA, FSCAI
Director, Hypertrophic Cardiomyopathy
Program, Director, Cardiac Catheterization
Laboratory, Division of Cardiology,
Westchester Medical Center, Associate
Professor of Medicine, New York Medical
College, Valhalla, New York, USA

JULIO A. PANZA, MD, FACC, FAHA
Chief, Division of Cardiology, Westchester
Medical Center, Professor of Medicine,
New York Medical College, Valhalla,
New York, USA

AUTHORS

ALLISON L. CIRINO, MS
Cardiovascular Division, Brigham and
Women's Hospital, Boston, Massachusetts,
USA

JOHN T. FALLON, MD, PhD
Director, Department of Clinical Laboratories
and Pathology, Westchester Medical Center,
Professor of Medicine and Pathology, Chair of
Pathology, New York Medical College,
Valhalla, New York, USA

MICHAEL A. FIFER, MD
Director, Hypertrophic Cardiomyopathy
Program, Massachusetts General Hospital,
Professor of Medicine, Harvard Medical
School, Boston, Massachusetts, USA

KATHERINE L. FISCHER, MSN, RN
Nurse Coordinator, Department of Cardiology,
OHSU Hypertrophic Cardiomyopathy Center,
Knight Cardiovascular Institute, Oregon Health
& Science University, Portland, Oregon, USA

ANTHON FUISZ, MD
Director of Advanced Cardiac Imaging,
Westchester Medical Center, Valhalla,
Wisconsin, USA

ALAN GASS, MD
Medical Director, Heart Transplant and
Mechanical Circulatory Support, Division of
Cardiology, Professor, Department of
Medicine, Westchester Medical Center, New
York Medical College, Valhalla, New York, USA

CHHAYA AGGARWAL GUPTA, MD
Attending, Advanced Heart Failure and
Cardiac Transplantation, Division of
Cardiology, Assistant Professor, Department
of Medicine, Westchester Medical Center,
New York Medical College, Valhalla, New York,
USA

STEPHEN B. HEITNER, MD, FACC
Director, Department of Cardiology, OHSU
Hypertrophic Cardiomyopathy Center, Knight
Cardiovascular Institute, Oregon Health &
Science University, Portland, Oregon, USA

CAROLYN Y. HO, MD
Cardiovascular Division, Brigham and
Women's Hospital, Boston, Massachusetts,
USA

SARAH HOSS, MD
University Health Network, Toronto, Ontario,
Canada

SEI IWAI, MD
Professor of Clinical Medicine, New York
Medical College, Director, Cardiac
Electrophysiology, Westchester Medical
Center Health System, Valhalla, New York,
USA

JASON T. JACOBSON, MD, FACC, FHRS
Associate Professor, Director, Complex
Arrhythmia Ablation Program, New York
Medical College, Westchester Medical Center,
Valhalla, New York, USA

GREGG M. LANIER, MD
Director, Pulmonary Hypertension Program,
Associate Director, Heart Failure, Westchester
Medical Center, Associate Professor of
Medicine, New York Medical College, Valhalla,
New York, USA

AVI LEVINE, MD
Attending, Advanced Heart Failure and Cardiac
Transplantation, Division of Cardiology,
Assistant Professor, Department of Medicine,
Westchester Medical Center, New York
Medical College, Valhalla, New York, USA

MATTHEW MARTINEZ, MD
Division of Cardiology, Lehigh Valley Health
Network, Allentown, Pennsylvania, USA

SRIHARI S. NAIDU, MD, FACC, FAHA, FSCAI
Director, Hypertrophic Cardiomyopathy
Program, Director, Cardiac Catheterization
Laboratory, Division of Cardiology,
Westchester Medical Center, Associate
Professor of Medicine, New York Medical
College, Valhalla, New York, USA

ANITA NGUYEN, MBBS
Department of Cardiovascular Surgery, Mayo
Clinic, Rochester, Minnesota, USA

JULIO A. PANZA, MD, FACC, FAHA
Chief, Division of Cardiology, Westchester
Medical Center, Professor of Medicine, New
York Medical College, Valhalla, New York, USA

HARRY RAKOWSKI, MD, FRCP, FACC, FASE
Professor of Medicine, University of Toronto,
Douglas Wigle Chair in HCM Research,
Director, Hypertrophic Cardiomyopathy Clinic,
Toronto General Hospital, University Health
Network, Toronto, Ontario, Canada

ABDALLAH SANAANI, MD
Attending Physician, Gunderson Health
System, La Crosse Campus, La Crosse,
Wisconsin, USA

HARTZELL V. SCHAFF, MD
Department of Cardiovascular Surgery, Mayo
Clinic, Rochester, Minnesota, USA

CHRISTINE E. SEIDMAN, MD
Cardiovascular Division, Brigham and
Women's Hospital, Department of Genetics,
Harvard Medical School, Boston,
Massachusetts, USA; Howard Hughes Medical
Institute, HHMI Investigator Program, Chevy
Chase, Maryland, USA

LYNNE K. WILLIAMS, MBBCh
Papworth Hospital NHS Foundation Trust,
Cambridge, United Kingdom

TIMOTHY C. WONG, MD, MS
Assistant Professor, Department of Medicine,
Division of Cardiology, University of Pittsburgh
School of Medicine, Director, UPMC
Hypertrophic Cardiomyopathy Center, UPMC
Heart and Vascular Institute, Pittsburgh,
Pennsylvania, USA

Contents

Historical Perspectives in the Evolution of Hypertrophic Cardiomyopathy   1

Julio A. Panza and Srihari S. Naidu

> Since the first anatomic description of hypertrophic cardiomyopathy (HCM) in 1958, significant advancements have expanded the understanding of this condition. At the same time, new imaging tools and treatment modalities have contributed to an ever-changing armamentarium for the assessment and treatment of patients with HCM. The historical perspective of HCM discovery and the progress made in the last several decades shed light on the road still ahead, which is expected to lead to better forms of treatment and perhaps even prevention of this, at times, devastating disease.

Echocardiography in the Diagnosis and Management of Hypertrophic Cardiomyopathy   11

Harry Rakowski, Sarah Hoss, and Lynne K. Williams

> Hypertrophic cardiomyopathy (HCM) is an inherited condition present in about 1/500 individuals with more than 1500 causative mutations identified in primarily 10 sarcomeric proteins. Although HCM is inherited in an autosomal dominant way, there is often incomplete penetrance and variable phenotype even with the same genotype. It is characterized by a degree of hypertrophy (usually asymmetric), that is, not due to another identifiable cause, as well as variable degrees of myocardial fibrosis and microvascular abnormalities.

Cardiac Magnetic Resonance for Diagnosis and Risk Stratification   27

Abdallah Sanaani and Anthon Fuisz

> Cardiac MRI (CMR) is an essential tool for the evaluation of the patient with hypertrophic cardiomyopathy (HCM). First, the accurate morphologic imaging and measures that are possible with CMR help to ascertain the diagnosis. Second, the tissue characterization that can be done with MRI helps to define the abnormalities in the myocardium and to identify areas of fibrosis that have been linked to increase risk of sudden cardiac death and heart failure. In addition, CMR can help distinguish HCM from similar disease processes.

Genetic Testing and Counseling for Hypertrophic Cardiomyopathy   35

Allison L. Cirino, Christine E. Seidman, and Carolyn Y. Ho

> Genetic testing has become more accessible and is increasingly being incorporated into the care of patients with hypertrophic cardiomyopathy. Genetic test results can help to refine diagnosis and distinguish at-risk relatives from those who are not at risk.

Hypertrophic cardiomyopathy is a heterogenous condition associated with a myriad of symptoms. Just as in other disease states, the aim of medical therapy is the alleviation of suffering, improvement of longevity, and the prevention of complications. This article focuses on the associated comorbidities seen in patients with hypertrophic cardiomyopathy, potential lifestyle interventions, and conventional medical treatments for symptomatic hypertrophic cardiomyopathy.

Patients with hypertrophic cardiomyopathy may present with a number of arrhythmias. Although not unique, arrhythmias in hypertrophic cardiomyopathy require management approaches that may differ from other populations. Standard permanent pacemaker indications can be seen, but unique applications and implantation considerations pertain to this population. Ventricular and supraventricular tachyarrhythmias may be experienced by patients with hypertrophic cardiomyopathy, treatment for which must be tailored to the hypertrophic cardiomyopathy substrate. In this article, permanent pacemaker indications, techniques and special considerations, and specific management issues of ventricular and supraventricular tachyarrhythmias in hypertrophic cardiomyopathy, are discussed.

Hypertrophic cardiomyopathy (HCM) is associated with an increased risk of sudden cardiac death (SCD), although perhaps not as significantly as previously believed. Given the heterogeneous nature of this disease entity, risk stratification of individuals with HCM remains challenging. The recent HCM risk-SCD prediction model seems to perform well in assessing individual SCD risk. Even though implantable cardiac defibrillators (ICDs) are effective in preventing SCD in patients at increased risk, the importance of shared decision making in deciding whether or not to undergo ICD implantation cannot be understated.

Hypertrophic cardiomyopathy affects 0.5% of the population. Advanced testing is considered, including cardiac catheterization, endomyocardial biopsy, and cardiopulmonary exercise testing. Right and left heart catheterization provides essential hemodynamic data, identifies patients who might benefit from septal reduction therapy, and assesses for comorbidities. Pathologic analysis reveals ventricular hypertrophy, myocardial disarray, and endocardial and interstitial fibrosis. Routine endomyocardial biopsy is not recommended unless other conditions that cause hypertrophy need to be ruled out. Cardiopulmonary exercise testing provides useful physiologic data, allows monitoring of the response to medication and surgical interventions, estimates prognosis, and guides referral for orthotopic heart transplantation.

Choice of Septal Reduction Therapies and Alcohol Septal Ablation

Michael A. Fifer

In patients with resting or provoked gradients and symptoms refractory to optimal medical therapy, alcohol septal ablation or surgical septal myectomy may be considered. Given the overall comparable outcomes after ablation and myectomy, there is, for many patients, equipoise between the two procedures. Septal ablation is performed with standard angioplasty guiding catheters, guidewires, and balloon catheters. In the Euro-ASA registry, NYHA functional class fell from 2.9 ± 0.5 to 1.6 ± 0.7 and gradient from 67 ± 36 to 16 ± 21 mm Hg at mean 3.9-year follow-up after septal ablation.

Surgical Myectomy: Subaortic, Midventricular, and Apical

Anita Nguyen and Hartzell V. Schaff

Surgical septal myectomy is the preferred method of septal reduction for most patients with obstructive hypertrophic cardiomyopathy whose symptoms do not respond to medical management. Transaortic extended septal myectomy has low operative mortality and provides durable relief of symptoms. Surgical treatment is possible for patients with less common phenotypes, such as complex long-segment septal hypertrophy, midventricular obstruction, or apical hypertrophic cardiomyopathy. For these anatomic subtypes, transapical myectomy can be used alone or combined with transaortic myectomy. This article describes both of these surgical techniques and discusses preoperative considerations and postoperative management for patients with hypertrophic cardiomyopathy.

Advanced Heart Failure Management and Transplantation

Avi Levine, Chhaya Aggarwal Gupta, and Alan Gass

Hypertrophic cardiomyopathy is a genetic heart disease with heterogeneous clinical features, including progression to advanced heart failure. The development of these symptoms can be related to outflow obstruction but in some patients reflects an underlying process of fibrosis and progressive ventricular dysfunction. For patients with end-stage disease, traditional heart failure therapies have not proved beneficial. As such, more advanced therapies, such as left ventricular assist device or cardiac transplantation, should be considered for these patients. Although left ventricular assist device support is used infrequently due to the restrictive physiology underlying hypertrophic cardiomyopathy, transplant represents an effective treatment, with encouraging long-term outcome data.

Novel Pharmacotherapy for Hypertrophic Cardiomyopathy

Timothy C. Wong and Matthew Martinez

Medical therapy for hypertrophic cardiomyopathy (HCM) has focused on minimizing the impact of symptoms due to left ventricular outflow tract obstruction and diastolic dysfunction. This article briefly discusses currently available therapy and focuses on both *clinically available medications* with novel applications for HCM as well as *novel medications* under development with specific indication for HCM. Finally, a brief summary of the current gaps and potential targets for pharmacotherapy is discussed.

CARDIOLOGY CLINICS

THE CLINICS ARE AVAILABLE ONLINE!
Access your subscription at:
www.theclinics.com

Preface

Hypertrophic Cardiomyopathy: Mastering the Multiple Facets of a Complex Disease

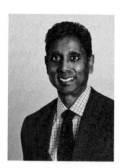
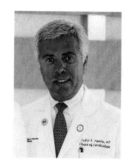

Srihari S. Naidu, MD, FACC, FAHA, FSCAI   Julio A. Panza, MD, FACC, FAHA

Editors

To study hypertrophic cardiomyopathy (HCM) and become a scholar on its diagnosis and treatment is not an easy task. On the one hand, it is a relatively rare cardiac condition, one to which most cardiologists are infrequently exposed in their daily clinical practice. On the other hand, it is a disease characterized by an enormous degree of variable presentations, such that virtually nothing about HCM is common to all patients who suffer from it. From the multiple causative genetic mutations to the extremely wide array of clinical manifestations, comprehending the full spectrum of HCM represents a difficult challenge, even to the most accomplished scientist or to the most astute clinician.

Accordingly, to face a patient with HCM, or even one suspected to have the disease, requires a thorough familiarity of every facet of clinical cardiology, from prevention and lifestyle modifications to the treatment of heart failure, including heart transplantation. Included within this wide range are the recognition and treatment of cardiac arrhythmias, knowledge about the means to diagnose and treat left ventricular outflow tract obstruction, methods for stratification regarding the risk of sudden cardiac death, and many other facets that make HCM arguably the most fascinating cardiac disease.

Perhaps because of the heterogeneity in the morphologic and clinical presentations, it may not be surprising that both the study and the understanding of HCM over the last several decades have included many disputes and controversies. *What is the appropriate name for a condition to which more than 50 terms have been applied? Is the pressure gradient across the left ventricular outflow tract indicative of real obstruction or simply artefactual? Is the gradient relief observed in some patients with right ventricular pacing a potential therapeutic tool or a sham intervention? What is the best treatment for obstruction refractory to medical therapy: surgical myectomy, or alcohol septal ablation? Is there HCM without hypertrophy?* Some of these, and several other, questions have been answered, and some remain in the realm of ongoing disagreements or uncertainties.

Undoubtedly, the efforts of innumerable scientists and clinical investigators have resulted in significant advances in our understanding of the multiple manifestations of HCM. Nevertheless, the most novel

Cardiol Clin 37 (2019) ix–x
https://doi.org/10.1016/j.ccl.2018.09.002
0733-8651/19/© 2018 Published by Elsevier Inc.

widely adopted treatment strategy, namely, alcohol septal ablation, was introduced nearly 25 years ago, with no new therapies developed in the current century. Hence, a gap of knowledge still remains, surely to be filled by the unrelenting progress of modern cardiovascular medicine.

Within this context, the present issue of *Cardiology Clinics* attempts to encapsulate every aspect of HCM in a comprehensive manner. Each author has made an effort to summarize the enormous amount of available material in articles that convey state-of-the-art knowledge in a didactic format. In addition, the totality of the work has been edited to ascertain that every aspect of HCM is addressed, avoiding unnecessary repetition of information. As a result, we believe this work will be of use to both the novice and the scholar.

Srihari S. Naidu, MD, FACC, FAHA, FSCAI
Hypertrophic Cardiomyopathy Center
Cardiac Catheterization Laboratory
Westchester Medical Center
New York Medical College
Macy Pavilion, Room 106
100 Woods Road
Valhalla, NY 10595, USA

Julio A. Panza, MD, FACC, FAHA
Westchester Medical Center
New York Medical College
Macy Pavilion, Room 100
100 Woods Road
Valhalla, NY 10595, USA

E-mail addresses:
srihari.naidu@wmchealth.org (S.S. Naidu)
julio.panza@wmchealth.org (J.A. Panza)

Historical Perspectives in the Evolution of Hypertrophic Cardiomyopathy

Julio A. Panza, MD*, Srihari S. Naidu, MD

KEYWORDS

- Hypertrophic cardiomyopathy • Septal myectomy • Genetics • Alcohol septal ablation
- Implantable cardioverter-defibrillator

KEY POINTS

- Physicians have postulated the existence of a disease characterized by syncope, sudden death, and a systolic murmur since the seventeenth century.
- The first anatomic description of hypertrophic cardiomyopathy (HCM) dates from 1958 by Dr Teare.
- The initial focus was on the obstructive form of HCM, hence the first medical (β-blockers) and surgical (septal myectomy) therapies were designed to address the dynamic outflow tract obstruction.
- Cardiac imaging, especially echocardiography, has contributed significantly to the understanding of HCM's presentation, its development, and the identification of different clinical and hemodynamic manifestations.
- Implantable cardioverter-defibrillators are currently the only therapy capable of altering the course of HCM by preventing sudden cardiac death caused by ventricular arrhythmias.

INTRODUCTION

Since the first description of the entity that was initially considered a possible cardiac tumor, 60 years have elapsed, resulting in significant advancements in the understanding and treatment of hypertrophic cardiomyopathy (HCM), a disease that has captivated the attention, and at times the imagination, of many clinicians and scientists. The history of the discovery of the disease, the multiple names it has received over the last 6 decades, the variable clinical presentations, and the significant advances in understanding the genetic basis for this condition are fascinating. In fact, the pathway toward the discovery of the disease has been presented as the model for scientific discovery, together with the proposal of 4 distinct and different phases that are logically linked.[1]

EVOLUTION OF KNOWLEDGE ABOUT HYPERTROPHIC CARDIOMYOPATHY

First Anatomic Description of Hypertrophic Cardiomyopathy

The British pathologist Robert Donald Teare[2] is usually credited with the discovery of the disease in a now classic citation from 1958, in which he reported 8 cases of young patients between the ages of 14 and 44 years, 7 of whom died suddenly. In an addendum to the same article, he briefly described a ninth patient, who was the brother of one of the patients previously mentioned; both he and his sister had died suddenly, thus establishing for the first time the familial nature of sudden death as part of the condition. The heart specimens showed asymmetric septal hypertrophy resembling a cardiac tumor, which he termed "a muscular hamartoma of the heart" and on

Disclosures: None.

Division of Cardiology, Westchester Medical Center, New York Medical College, 100 Woods Road, Macy Pavilion, Suite 11, Valhalla, NY 10595, USA

* Corresponding author.

E-mail address: julio.panza@wmchealth.org

Cardiol Clin 37 (2019) 1–10

https://doi.org/10.1016/j.ccl.2018.08.001

histology he showed, for the first time, the now typically recognized and pathognomonic "disorganized arrangement of muscle bundles associated with hypertrophy of individual muscle fibers and their nuclei." It is now known that, although there are certain characteristic features of the heart specimens that are considered typical of HCM, no single finding is present in all hearts.[3] For example, the traditional hallmark of the disease, namely asymmetric septal hypertrophy, was only present in about two-thirds of 230 cases reviewed by Dr William C. Roberts[4] in the 50-year span between 1959 and 2008.

Prehistory of Hypertrophic Cardiomyopathy

Although Teare's[2] is appropriately recognized as the first description of a condition characterized by asymmetric septal hypertrophy, myocardial disarray on histology, and sudden death in the same family, it is clear that the observation of enlarged hearts in patients dying suddenly had puzzled physicians for at least 3 centuries. In the scholarly article in which Coats and Hollman[5] reviewed the early history of HCM, they quote Théophile Bonet (1620–1689), a Swiss physician who had published a large collection of postmortem specimens and John Baptiste Morgagni (1682–1771), a pathologist who refined Bonet's work. Bonet first wrote: "A coachman died suddenly in his carriage whose heart was larger than that of any bullock, another sudden death of a heart far exceeding its natural bulk." Morgagni later recalled another case: "Often troubled with palpitations particularly in the night, an oppressive pain in the chest, sometimes was afraid of a swooning and at other times of suffocation, the circulation of the blood being obstructed from the left ventricle into the artery." Coats and Hollman[5] present this as the first evidence of the recognition of left ventricular outflow tract obstruction in HCM.

Notwithstanding these very early and other subsequent[6–9] reports of the association between enlarged hearts, symptoms (chest pain, breathlessness, and syncope [swooning]) and sudden cardiac death, it is appropriate to credit Teare[2] as the first to describe the characteristic morphologic pattern of the disease in patients who had died suddenly, and hence to establish HCM as a distinct cardiac disease entity. Teare and his colleagues[10,11] also described the familial pattern of the disease and even its pathophysiologic hallmark of obstruction to left ventricular outflow in subsequent publications from 1960. Further, what is remarkable about Teare's[2] original article is that, in the description of 8 cases, he encapsulated most of the clinical, pathologic, and natural history features of HCM that are now recognized as hallmarks of this condition.

Early Advances in Understanding Hypertrophic Cardiomyopathy

It is important to recognize that, around this time, several other groups around the world reported the existence of the same pathologic features in different families[10–19] in a quintessential example of simultaneous scientific discovery, each investigator contributing to the collective understanding of the disease. By 1960, the medical literature had been populated by multiple descriptions of a discrete disease entity characterized by a mendelian pattern of inheritance, asymmetric left ventricular hypertrophy, nonanatomic obstruction to left ventricular outflow, myocardial disarray on histology, symptoms consistent with myocardial ischemia and heart failure, and sudden death as a common mechanism of demise.

Focus on Dynamic Subaortic Obstruction

It is clear that all reports from the late 1950s and early 1960s exclusively focused on the obstructive form of the disease. Despite these sagacious early reports, it was not until 1964 that the obstructive form of HCM was described in extensive detail by Dr Eugene Braunwald and colleagues[20] working at the National Institutes of Health (NIH) in Bethesda, Maryland. In 3 articles covering 213 pages published as an American Heart Association monograph, Braunwald and colleagues,[20] Morrow and colleagues,[21] and Pierce and colleagues[22] coined the term idiopathic hypertrophic subaortic stenosis (IHSS; still in use by some clinicians) describing virtually all aspects of the disease, including the putative mechanism of obstruction and its pharmacologic and operative treatment. By the mid-1960s, the abnormal systolic anterior motion (SAM) of the mitral valve with its resultant mitral regurgitation were described on angiography, unifying the different theories regarding the mechanism and hemodynamic consequences of left ventricular outflow tract obstruction,[23,24] and, by the late 1960s, the medical literature saw the first noninvasive description of SAM using ultrasound waves.[25]

The Revolution of Echocardiography

The development of M-mode echocardiography in the 1970s allowed the noninvasive assessment of the pathophysiology of obstructive HCM, including the description of the systolic semiclosure of the aortic valve as a consequence of the more proximal impediment to left ventricular outflow. At the same time, it allowed the realization that SAM was not present in all patients with HCM, whereas asymmetric septal hypertrophy was.[26] This observation, also made at the NIH after the departure of Dr Braunwald, led to discovery of the more frequent nonobstructive form and to the proposal of the term asymmetric septal hypertrophy (ASH) as the more appropriate name for the disease. To quote Henry and colleagues[26]: "Our results indicate that it is possible to identify patients with IHSS on the basis of the echocardiographic demonstration of asymmetric septal hypertrophy. This abnormality is independent of the existence of a left ventricular outflow tract gradient" and "We suggest that a more appropriate term for this disease entity is asymmetric septal hypertrophy or ASH." Subsequently, with the advent of two-dimensional echocardiography, it was evident that the distribution of hypertrophy is not always consistent with ASH. Maron and colleagues[27] were the first to describe the different patterns of hypertrophy in different segments of the left ventricle; others also described unusual patterns and their significance.[28,29]

In the late 1980s, the advent of Doppler echocardiography allowed hemodynamic assessment to be obtained noninvasively and quantitative measurements of the pressure gradient across the left ventricular outflow tract using continuous-wave Doppler were validated against the invasive measurements obtained in the catheterization laboratory.[30,31] This important development permitted investigators to question the proposal that increased velocities across the outflow tract were causative in the generation of SAM.[32] This alternative view has also been supported by the experimental demonstration that displacement of the papillary muscles can lead to SAM and dynamic subaortic obstruction.[33] Further, primary abnormalities of the mitral valve are common among patients with obstructive HCM, suggesting that the initial hypothesis of SAM solely caused by Venturi forces created by vigorous ejection of blood through the outflow tract may have been an oversimplification of the pathophysiology and anatomic variability intrinsic to dynamic obstruction in this condition. It became clear that abnormalities of the mitral valve itself contribute causally to the presence and pattern of dynamic obstruction.[34–36] In addition, Doppler echocardiography also allowed the assessment of diastolic function using pulsed-wave Doppler,[37] Doppler tissue imaging,[38] and (more recently) strain imaging.[39]

The advances in imaging understandably led to significant progress in the knowledge of the disease process. Thus, despite the initial focus on the presence and mechanism of dynamic obstruction, most patients were shown to have no significant resting obstruction,[40] although, in a significant number, the gradient can be provoked in the noninvasive laboratory.[41] The availability of echocardiograms in children followed longitudinally allowed the observation that the disease can develop de novo during childhood and adolescence, usually temporally associated to periods of rapid body growth spurts.[42] Further, even the dynamic left ventricular outflow tract obstruction can also develop during young life.[43] Later, it was shown that left ventricular hypertrophy can also develop de novo in the fourth and even the fifth decade of life in patients with certain genetic mutations.[44]

Understanding the Genetics Background of Hypertrophic Cardiomyopathy

The familial pattern of inheritance of HCM was first suggested in the original publication by Teare[2] and demonstrated in the early descriptions of the disease. That there are extremely variable morphologic presentations within the same genotypic background was evident soon after two-dimensional echocardiography permitted the noninvasive assessment of the condition in multiple members of the same family.[45] However, it was not until 1990 that the first evidence of the genetic basis of the disease was unveiled with the discovery of a disease-causing mutation in the cardiac beta-myosin heavy chain.[46] Shortly after, the same group of investigators reported a different missense mutation in the beta-myosin heavy chain gene in the family originally reported by Teare and colleagues,[47] in yet another interesting twist in the history of HCM discovery. In the ensuing decade, mutations have been discovered in multiple genes encoding for many sarcomeric proteins, including troponin I, troponin T, troponin C, myosin-binding protein-C, α-tropomyosin, essential myosin light chain, titin, actin, and α-cardiac myosin heavy chain.[48] Genotype-phenotype correlations have been described in HCM[49]; however, a genetic basis is found in only about a third of patients with documented HCM[50] and the phenotypic variability of the disease remains perplexing. Perhaps the most puzzling presentation is the one without left ventricular hypertrophy in a person with known genetic mutation. This genotype-positive, phenotype-negative clinical scenario,[51] still of undefined significance, constitutes the paradox of HCM without hypertrophy, an apparent contradiction in terms.

Thus, the concept of HCM has evolved significantly from the one initially offered by Teare[2] in

1958. From a disease initially described as tumor-like hypertrophy of the interventricular septum, followed by the challenge of understanding the pathophysiology of obstruction to left ventricular outflow without anatomic impediment, and continuing with the discovery of the genetic basis for the disease, the first 60 years have brought many changes in how clinicians understand and even define HCM. However, despite all these advances, a unifying concept of HCM is still missing: is it 1 disease with different genetic backgrounds or is it several genetic abnormalities sharing certain phenotypic expressions? It is only logical to expect that knowledge of HCM will continue to evolve and expand in the decades to come.

EVOLUTION IN THE ASSESSMENT OF PATIENTS WITH HYPERTROPHIC CARDIOMYOPATHY
Clinical Examination

In 1957 (ie, 1 year before the anatomic description by Teare[2]) Paul Wood recognized the clinical signs of obstructive HCM in a letter written after 4 patients were operated for aortic stenosis without the finding of anatomic obstruction at the level of the aortic valve. In a communication referring to a specific patient he had evaluated, Wood wrote "I think I know what this is now, and we call it functional muscular subvalvar aortic stenosis. It is due to gross hypertrophy of the outflow tract of the left ventricle for reasons we still do not understand. The muscle gets so thick that it tends to obstruct itself and so cause the outflow tract murmur and thrill." It is amazing that Wood was able to describe a disease that he had not seen. Further, he went on to state "Perhaps I could see Mrs. X again in a year's time. The prognosis, I am afraid, is rather guarded although I gave her no indication of that."[52] This communication clearly constitutes the earliest and most astute description of the disease using just the physical examination.

Cardiac Catheterization

Because the disease was initially defined by the presence of subaortic obstruction, the initial assessment of the condition was determined by the need to demonstrate the difference from the better known valvular aortic stenosis. Hence, cardiac catheterization became a necessary tool for the evaluation of the presence, location, and physiology of the intraventricular gradient. At the NIH, Brockenbrough and colleagues[53] pioneered this form of evaluation, including the now classic description of the decrease in stroke volume and systemic blood pressure in the beat that follows the provocation of a premature ventricular contraction, giving rise to the sign that carries their name. In addition, cardiac catheterization permitted the dynamic visualization of the left ventricular cavity and the description of the so-called ballerina-slip appearance on ventriculography at end-systole.[54]

Noninvasive Imaging: Echocardiography

The development of echocardiography has been the most important step forward for the assessment of patients with HCM. Modern echocardiography remains the most relevant study to be performed in the evaluation of patients with known or suspected HCM. At the same time, the evolution of echocardiography parallels the evolution in the understanding of the HCM disease process. As limited as M-mode echocardiography seems to be compared with other current imaging modalities, it was this method that first allowed the real-time assessment of the role of the mitral valve in the genesis of the subaortic obstruction,[25] its response to provocation maneuvers and relief with β-blockers,[55] and later even a noninvasive and repeatable quantitative estimation of the outflow tract gradient.[56,57] Further, with M-mode echocardiography it became clear that not all patients with HCM had outflow tract obstruction and that ASH was a hallmark of the disease, hence establishing for the first time the basis for diagnosing the disease noninvasively.[26,58]

Notwithstanding these important contributions of M-mode echocardiography, the cardiac examination allowed by this technique is limited to only a few segments of the left ventricle. Therefore, it was not until two-dimensional echocardiography came to the clinical arena that the ability to detect areas of abnormally thick myocardium over the entire left ventricular wall became possible. Thus, it became clear that ASH was not an appropriate name for the disease, because areas other than the anterior ventricular septum may be involved, thus not resulting in the abnormally increased septal/free-wall ratio that M-mode echocardiography can detect.[27] Accordingly, two-dimensional echocardiography quickly became, and has remained, the essential tool for the assessment of patients with HCM and for the screening of their relatives. In addition to the demonstration of usual and unusual forms of distribution of left ventricular hypertrophy, echocardiography contributed importantly to the description of the associated abnormalities of the mitral valve,[59] including the coexistence of mitral valve prolapse in some patients,[60] and the different patterns of obstruction to left ventricular outflow.[33–36] The advent of Doppler echocardiography in the 1980s allowed the noninvasive assessment of the presence and magnitude of the outflow tract gradient with the same accuracy as the invasive cardiac catheterization,[31] thus rendering this latter method unnecessary for this purpose. Moreover, the combination of Doppler with provocation maneuvers established that a large proportion of patients with HCM have the obstructive form of the disease.[41] Overall, cardiac ultrasonography has unarguably been the most insightful and impactful development in the assessment of patients with HCM.

Cardiac Magnetic Resonance

The most advanced form of imaging, particularly germane to patients with HCM, is cardiac magnetic resonance (CMR). Although CMR imaging was developed in the 1980s, it was not until the first decade of the twenty-first century that its utility for the assessment of patients with HCM was fully realized.[61,62] Because of its superior spatial resolution, and the high-quality images that result from the sharp contrast between the myocardial border, the blood pool, and the surrounding structures, CMR has added significantly to the assessment of patients with HCM. One the most notable contributions of CMR is the ability to clearly define hypertrophy in areas of the left ventricle for which the echocardiographic assessment may be suboptimal in certain patients, such as those with poor ultrasonography windows. These areas include the left ventricular apex, hence the greater ability of CMR, compared with echocardiography, to identify left ventricular apical aneurysms.[63] In addition, the use of gadolinium allows the identification of myocardial fibrosis using the late gadolinium enhancement method. This technique has prognostic implications, because it has been shown that the presence of fibrosis, measured by CMR, extending for greater than 15% of the myocardial mass conveys an increased risk of sudden death[64,65] and has become one of the evolving criteria for consideration of implantable cardioverter-defibrillator (ICD).

Other Nonimaging Methods

In addition to imaging of the left ventricle, other noninvasive tests play an important role in the assessment of HCM, including ambulatory electrocardiogram monitoring, because it allows the identification of episodes of nonsustained ventricular tachycardia during daily life, which may have negative prognostic implications.[66,67] In addition, the conventional exercise stress test, particularly when combined with meticulous measurements of the blood pressure response, also has prognostic value, because it has been shown that a

decrease in systolic blood pressure of more than 20 mm Hg is associated with increased risk of sudden death.[68,69]

EVOLUTION IN THE TREATMENT OF HYPERTROPHIC CARDIOMYOPATHY
Medical Therapy

Of significant interest is that all forms of therapy in HCM have been developed in response to observations about the pathophysiology or clinical course of the disease. β-blockers were the first drugs used to relieve symptoms because of their negative inotropic properties. The hypothesis that negative inotropic agents may be beneficial in obstructive HCM stemmed from the observations that digitalis[70] and isoproterenol[71] induced an increase in the dynamic left ventricular outflow tract gradient. This phenomenon, different from that observed in patients with valvular aortic stenosis, led to the concept that blocking the beta receptors would produce the opposite effect. A novel (at the time) drug named Nethalide was the first βblocker used by Braunwald and colleagues[72] to prove this hypothesis at the NIH in the early 1960s. Subsequently, the long-term effect of β-blockers was shown[73] and these drugs remain as the first-line agents in patients with HCM to relieve symptoms.[74] Other negative inotropic drugs were later developed in the 1980s and are currently in use as second-line agents. These drugs include the calcium channel blocker verapamil[75,76] and the type Ia antiarrhythmic agent disopyramide.[77,78]

Surgical Myectomy

Although medical therapy is the initial form of treatment in HCM, as it is in virtually every cardiovascular disease, surgical myectomy was the first form of therapy ever conceived and performed for this condition, largely because of the focus on obstruction to left ventricular outflow in the first years of disease discovery. The first myectomy in obstructive HCM was performed in London by W.P. Cleland in 1958[5,11] on a patient suspected to have subaortic obstruction based on the preoperative demonstration of a gradient between the left ventricle and the aorta without aortic valve calcification. According to Coats and Hollman,[5] the patient was found to have no gradient in the operating room. The surgeon was initially reluctant to proceed, but the cardiologist who had measured the gradient urged him to open the ascending aorta, confirm the normal aortic valve and the extensively hypertrophied interventricular septum, and to excise part of the abnormal tissue. Despite these early attempts, the credit for pioneering surgical myectomy belongs to Dr A.G.

Morrow, the chief surgeon at the NIH in Bethesda, who designed the operation based on other surgical techniques to relieve muscular obstruction.[79–81] The surgical technique that carries his name has been modified by others but still remains the most effective technique for the long-term relief of dynamic subaortic obstruction and its associated symptoms. In addition, surgical myectomy may restore the life expectancy of patients with HCM to that of the general population.[82] As another fascinating aspect of HCM history, it is worth noting that Dr Morrow himself had obstructive HCM and died of its complications.[83] More recently, surgical techniques involving muscle resection have been developed for patients with other forms of HCM, including midventricular obstruction,[84] apical aneurysms,[85] and even apical HCM without obstruction.[86]

Alcohol Septal Ablation

In the mid-1990s, the technique of septal reduction with injection of alcohol was first developed[87] and, since then, many centers have established the long-term efficacy and usefulness of this method.[88] However, controversy still exists about the relative merits of this therapy compared with the conventional surgical myectomy, despite similar outcomes with both forms of treatment.[89–91] In general, the surgical myectomy is considered the gold-standard form of treatment for sustained relief of symptoms caused by obstructive HCM. Transcatheter mitral valve plication has recently been proposed as another form of nonsurgical intervention for the relief of outflow tract obstruction.[92]

Dual-Chamber Pacing

The concept of pacemaker-induced dyssynchrony led to the development of right ventricular pacing as a potential form of treatment of obstructive HCM. Initial reports from the NIH suggested promising results.[93,94] However, a small randomized trial that enrolled a total of 48 patients showed that the symptomatic relief was not different from that observed with a sham procedure.[95] Whether dual-chamber pacing may benefit a subset of patients with obstructive HCM remains to be determined. Presently, permanent pacing as primary treatment of obstruction is not recommended unless patients are suboptimal candidates for septal reduction therapy or have a dual-chamber device implanted for other indications.[74]

Implantable Cardioverter-Defibrillator

It must be noted that all forms of therapy summarized earlier are only indicated for the relief of symptoms. In contradistinction, implantation of ICDs has been shown to forestall episodes of sudden death caused by ventricular arrhythmias[96] and thus ICDs are currently the only form of therapy indicated to improve the survival of patients with HCM, even in the absence of symptoms. Because of the potential problems associated with inappropriate firing and other device complications, only patients at high risk of sudden death are eligible for ICD placement.[74] To this end, a risk score calculator has been developed to help determine the appropriateness of ICD implantation in individual patients.[97] The score predicts the 5-year risk of sudden cardiac death based on known factors associated with increased risk, including age, extent of left ventricular hypertrophy, left atrial size, outflow tract gradient, family history of sudden death, nonsustained ventricular tachycardia, and unexplained syncope.

Preventing Hypertrophic Cardiomyopathy?

Finally, although prevention of HCM does not seem a priori to be a plausible concept, investigators have recently reported the correction of a pathogenic mutation in human embryos with the inherited genetic abnormality.[98] Whether this important scientific discovery can one day be translated into the clinical arena is part of the future of HCM treatment.

SUMMARY

As described in this article, the progress made over the last several decades in the understanding of HCM, and the resulting improved approach to the assessment and treatment of patients with HCM has been nothing short of astonishing. Reflecting on the 60 years since the first anatomic description of the disease, it is inevitable to conclude that the decades ahead will bring an even greater gain in the knowledge of this condition and its extremely variable presentations. It is therefore expected that the future will bring new and improved forms of treatment, particularly to address the most devastating presentations of HCM.

REFERENCES

1. Adelman H, Adelman A. The logic of discovery: a case study of hypertrophic cardiomyopathy. Acta Biotheor 1977;26:39–58.
2. Teare D. Asymmetrical hypertrophy of the heart in young adults. Br Heart J 1958;20:1–8.
3. Roberts CS, Roberts WC. Morphologic features of hypertrophic cardiomyopathy. In: Zipes DP,

Rowlands DJ, editors. Progress in cardiology. Philadelphia: Lea & Ferbirger; 1989. p. 3–32.

4. Roberts WC. Fifty years of hypertrophic cardiomyopathy. Am J Cardiol 2009;103:431–4.

5. Coats CJ, Hollman A. Hypertrophic cardiomyopathy: lessons from history. Heart 2008;94:1258–63.

6. Evans W. Familial cardiomegaly. Br Heart J 1949;11: 68–82.

7. Addarii F, Mahaim L, Winston M. Nouvelles recherches sur le "bloc bilateral manqué". Cardiologica 1946;11:36.

8. Davies LG. A familial heart disease. Br Heart J 1952; 14:206–12.

9. Gaunt R, Lecutier M. Familial cardiomegaly. Br Heart J 1956;18:251–8.

10. Hollman A, Goodwin JF, Teare D, et al. A family with obstructive cardiomyopathy. Br Heart J 1960;22:449–56.

11. Goodwin JF, Hollman A, Cleland WP, et al. Obstructive cardiomyopathy simulating aortic stenosis. Br Heart J 1960;22:403–14.

12. Brock R, Fleming PR. Aortic subvalvar stenosis; a report of 5 cases diagnosed during life. Guys Hosp Rep 1956;105:391–408.

13. Brock R. Functional obstruction of the left ventricle; acquired aortic subvalvar stenosis. Guys Hosp Rep 1957;106:221–38.

14. Bercu BA, Diettert GA, Danforth WH, et al. Pseudoaortic stenosis produced by ventricular hypertrophy. Am J Med 1958;25:814–8.

15. Morrow AG, Braunwald E. Functional aortic stenosis; a malformation characterized by resistance to left ventricular outflow without anatomic obstruction. Circulation 1959;20:181–9.

16. Wigle ED, Heimbecker RO, Gunton RW. Idiopathic ventricular septal hypertrophy causing muscular subaortic stenosis. Circulation 1962;26:325–40.

17. Braunwald E, Morrow AG, Cornell WP, et al. Idiopathic hypertrophic subaortic stenosis. Clinical, hemodynamic and angiographic manifestations. Am J Med 1960;29:924–5.

18. Brent LB, Aburano A, Fisher DL, et al. Familial muscular subaortic stenosis: an unrecognized form of "idiopathic heart diseases", with clinical and autopsy observations. Circulation 1960;21:167–80.

19. Pare JA, Fraser RG, Pirozynski WJ, et al. Hereditary cardiovascular dysplasia. A form of familial cardiomyopathy. Am J Med 1961;31:37–62.

20. Braunwald E, Lambrew CT, Rockoff SD, et al. A description of the disease based upon an analysis of 64 patients. Am Heart Assoc Monogr 1964;10: IV3–119.

21. Morrow AG, Lambrew CT, Braunwald E. Operative treatment and the results of pre- and postoperative hemodynamic evaluations. Am Heart Assoc Monogr 1964;10:IV120–51.

22. Pierce GE, Morrow AG, Braunwald E. Intraoperative studies of the mechanism of obstruction and its hemodynamic consequences. Am Heart Assoc Monogr 1964;10:IV152–213.

23. Fix P, Moberg A, Soederberg H, et al. Muscular subvalvular aortic stenosis; abnormal anterior mitral leaflet possibly the primary factor. Acta Radiol Diagn (Stockh) 1964;2:177–93.

24. Dinsmore RE, Sanders CA, Harthorne JW. Mitral regurgitation in idiopathic hypertrophic subaortic stenosis. N Engl J Med 1966;275:1225–8.

25. Shah PM, Gramiak R, Kramer DH. Ultrasound localization of left ventricular outflow obstruction in hypertrophic obstructive cardiomyopathy. Circulation 1969;40:3–11.

26. Henry WL, Clark CE, Epstein SE. Asymmetric septal hypertrophy. Echocardiographic identification of the pathognomonic anatomic abnormality of IHSS. Circulation 1973;47:225–33.

27. Maron BJ, Gottdiener JS, Epstein SE. Patterns and significance of distribution of left ventricular hypertrophy in hypertrophic cardiomyopathy. Am J Cardiol 1981;48:418–28.

28. Shapiro LM, McKenna WJ. Distribution of left ventricular hypertrophy in hypertrophic cardiomyopathy: a two-dimensional echocardiographic study. J Am Coll Cardiol 1983;2:437–44.

29. Wigle ED, Sasson Z, Henderson MA, et al. Hypertrophic cardiomyopathy. The importance of the site and the extent of hypertrophy. A review. Prog Cardiovasc Dis 1985;28:1–83.

30. Sasson Z, Yock PG, Hatle LK, et al. Doppler echocardiographic determination of the pressure gradient in hypertrophic cardiomyopathy. J Am Coll Cardiol 1988;11:752–6.

31. Panza JA, Petrone RK, Fananapazir L, et al. Utility of continuous wave Doppler echocardiography in the noninvasive assessment of left ventricular outflow tract pressure gradient in patients with hypertrophic cardiomyopathy. J Am Coll Cardiol 1992;19:91–9.

32. Sherrid MV, Gunsburg DZ, Moldenhauer S, et al. Systolic anterior motion begins at low left ventricular outflow tract velocity in obstructive hypertrophic cardiomyopathy. J Am Coll Cardiol 2000;36:1344–54.

33. Levine RA, Vlahakes GJ, Lefebvre X, et al. Papillary muscle displacement causes systolic anterior motion of the mitral valve. Experimental validation and insights into the mechanism of subaortic obstruction. Circulation 1995;91:1189–95.

34. Maron BJ, Harding AM, Spirito P, et al. Systolic anterior motion of the posterior mitral leaflet: a previously unrecognized cause of dynamic subaortic obstruction in patients with hypertrophic cardiomyopathy. Circulation 1983;68:282–93.

35. Klues HG, Roberts WC, Maron BJ. Anomalous insertion of papillary muscle directly into anterior mitral leaflet in hypertrophic cardiomyopathy. Significance in producing left ventricular outflow obstruction. Circulation 1991;84:1188–97.

36. Klues HG, Roberts WC, Maron BJ. Morphological determinants of echocardiographic patterns of mitral valve systolic anterior motion in obstructive hypertrophic cardiomyopathy. Circulation 1993;87: 1570–9.

37. Maron BJ, Spirito P, Green KJ, et al. Noninvasive assessment of left ventricular diastolic function by pulsed Doppler echocardiography in patients with hypertrophic cardiomyopathy. J Am Coll Cardiol 1987;10:733–42.

38. Geske JB, Sorajja P, Nishimura RA, et al. Evaluation of left ventricular filling pressures by Doppler echocardiography in patients with hypertrophic cardiomyopathy: correlation with direct left atrial pressure measurement at cardiac catheterization. Circulation 2007;116:2702–8.

39. Chen S, Yuan J, Qiao S, et al. Evaluation of left ventricular diastolic function by global strain rate imaging in patients with obstructive hypertrophic cardiomyopathy: a simultaneous speckle tracking echocardiography and cardiac catheterization study. Echocardiography 2014;31:615–22.

40. Maron BJ, Bonow RO, Cannon RO 3rd, et al. Hypertrophic cardiomyopathy. Interrelations of clinical manifestations, pathophysiology, and therapy (2). N Engl J Med 1987;316:844–52.

41. Maron MS, Olivotto I, Zenovich AG, et al. Hypertrophic cardiomyopathy is predominantly a disease of left ventricular outflow tract obstruction. Circulation 2006;114:2232–9.

42. Maron BJ, Spirito P, Wesley Y, et al. Development and progression of left ventricular hypertrophy in children with hypertrophic cardiomyopathy. N Engl J Med 1986;315:610–4.

43. Panza JA, Maris TJ, Maron BJ. Development and determinants of dynamic obstruction to left ventricular outflow in young patients with hypertrophic cardiomyopathy. Circulation 1992;85: 1398–405.

44. Maron BJ, Niimura H, Casey SA, et al. Development of left ventricular hypertrophy in adults in hypertrophic cardiomyopathy caused by cardiac myosin-binding protein C gene mutations. J Am Coll Cardiol 2001;38:315–21.

45. Ciró E, Nichols PF 3rd, Maron BJ. Heterogeneous morphologic expression of genetically transmitted hypertrophic cardiomyopathy. Two-dimensional echocardiographic analysis. Circulation 1983;67: 1227–33.

46. Geisterfer-Lowrance AA, Kass S, Tanigawa G, et al. A molecular basis for familial hypertrophic cardiomyopathy: a beta cardiac myosin heavy chain gene missense mutation. Cell 1990;62:999–1006.

47. Watkins H, Seidman CE, MacRae C, et al. Progress in familial hypertrophic cardiomyopathy: molecular genetic analyses in the original family studied by Teare. Br Heart 1992;67:34–8.

48. Keren A, Syrris P, McKenna WJ. Hypertrophic cardiomyopathy: the genetic determinants of clinical disease expression. Nat Clin Pract Cardiovasc Med 2008;5:158–68.

49. Marian AJ. Pathogenesis of diverse clinical and pathological phenotypes in hypertrophic cardiomyopathy. Lancet 2000;355:58–60.

50. Bos JM, Will ML, Gersh BJ, et al. Characterization of a phenotype-based genetic test prediction score for unrelated patients with hypertrophic cardiomyopathy. Mayo Clin Proc 2014;89:727–37.

51. Varnava A, Baboonian C, Davison F, et al. A new mutation of the cardiac troponin T gene causing familial hypertrophic cardiomyopathy without left ventricular hypertrophy. Heart 1999;82:621–4.

52. Somerville J. Paul Wood Lecture. The master's legacy: the first Paul Wood Lecture. Heart 1998;80: 612–8.

53. Brockenbrough EC, Braunwald E, Morrow AG. A hemodynamic technic for the detection of hypertrophic subaortic stenosis. Circulation 1961;23: 189–94.

54. Simon AL, Ross J Jr, Gault JH. Angiographic anatomy of the left ventricle and mitral valve in idiopathic hypertrophic subaortic stenosis. Circulation 1967; 36:852–67.

55. Popp RL, Harrison DC. Ultrasound in the diagnosis and evaluation of therapy of idiopathic hypertrophic subaortic stenosis. Circulation 1969;40: 905–14.

56. Henry WL, Clark CE, Glancy DL, et al. Echocardiographic measurement of the left ventricular outflow gradient in idiopathic hypertrophic subaortic stenosis. N Engl J Med 1973;288:989–93.

57. Pollick C, Rakowski H, Wigle ED. Muscular subaortic stenosis: the quantitative relationship between systolic anterior motion and the pressure gradient. Circulation 1984;69:43–9.

58. Abbasi AS, MacAlpin RN, Eber LM, et al. Echocardiographic diagnosis of idiopathic hypertrophic cardiomyopathy without outflow obstruction. Circulation 1972;46:897–904.

59. Klues HG, Proschan MA, Dollar AL, et al. Echocardiographic assessment of mitral valve size in obstructive hypertrophic cardiomyopathy. Anatomic validation from mitral valve specimen. Circulation 1993;88:548–55.

60. Panza JA, Maron BJ. Simultaneous occurrence of mitral valve prolapse and systolic anterior motion in hypertrophic cardiomyopathy. Am J Cardiol 1991;67:404–10.

61. Rickers C, Wilke NM, Jerosch-Herold M, et al. Utility of cardiac magnetic resonance imaging in the diagnosis of hypertrophic cardiomyopathy. Circulation 2005;112:855–61.

62. Olivotto I, Maron MS, Autore C, et al. Assessment and significance of left ventricular mass by

cardiovascular magnetic resonance in hypertrophic cardiomyopathy. J Am Coll Cardiol 2008;52: 559–66.

63. Maron MS, Finley JJ, Bos JM, et al. Prevalence, clinical significance, and natural history of left ventricular apical aneurysms in hypertrophic cardiomyopathy. Circulation 2008;118:1541–9.

64. Chan RH, Maron BJ, Olivotto I, et al. Prognostic value of quantitative contrast-enhanced cardiovascular magnetic resonance for the evaluation of sudden death risk in patients with hypertrophic cardiomyopathy. Circulation 2014;130:484–95.

65. Maron MS, Maron BJ. Clinical impact of contemporary cardiovascular magnetic resonance imaging in hypertrophic cardiomyopathy. Circulation 2015; 132:292–8.

66. Maron BJ, Savage DD, Wolfson JK, et al. Prognostic significance of 24-hour ambulatory electrocardiographic monitoring in patients with hypertrophic cardiomyopathy: a prospective study. Am J Cardiol 1981;48:252–7.

67. Monserrat L, Elliott PM, Gimeno JR, et al. Non-sustained ventricular tachycardia in hypertrophic cardiomyopathy: an independent marker of sudden death risk in young patients. J Am Coll Cardiol 2003;42:873–9.

68. Sadoul N, Prasad K, Elliott PM, et al. Prospective prognostic assessment of blood pressure response during exercise in patients with hypertrophic cardiomyopathy. Circulation 1997;96:2987–91.

69. Olivotto I, Maron BJ, Montereggi A, et al. Prognostic value of systemic blood pressure response during exercise in a community-based patient population with hypertrophic cardiomyopathy. J Am Coll Cardiol 1999;33:2044–51.

70. Braunwald E, Brockenbrough EC, Frye RL. Studies on digitalis. V. Comparison of the effects of ouabain on left ventricular dynamics in valvular aortic stenosis and hypertrophic subaortic stenosis. Circulation 1962;26:166–73.

71. Braunwald E, Ebert PA. Hemodynamic alterations in idiopathic hypertrophic subaortic stenosis induced by sympathomimetic drugs. Am J Cardiol 1962;10: 489–95.

72. Harrison DC, Braunwald E, Glick G, et al. Effects of beta adrenergic blockade on the circulation, with particular reference to observations in patients with hypertrophic subaortic stenosis. Circulation 1964; 29:84–98.

73. Stenson RE, Flamm MD Jr, Harrison DC, et al. Hypertrophic subaortic stenosis: clinical hemodynamic effects of long-term propranolol therapy. Am J Cardiol 1973;31:763–73.

74. Gersh BJ, Maron BJ, Bonow RO, et al. 2011 ACCF/ AHA guideline for the diagnosis and treatment of hypertrophic cardiomyopathy: a report of the American College of Cardiology Foundation/American Heart Association Task Force on Practice Guidelines. J Am Coll Cardiol 2011;58:e212–60.

75. Rosing DR, Kent KM, Borer JS, et al. Verapamil therapy: a new approach to the pharmacologic treatment of hypertrophic cardiomyopathy, I: hemodynamic effects. Circulation 1979;60:1201–7.

76. Rosing DR, Condit JR, Maron BJ, et al. Verapamil therapy: a new approach to the pharmacologic treatment of hypertrophic cardiomyopathy, III: effects of long-term administration. Am J Cardiol 1981;48:545–53.

77. Pollick C. Muscular subaortic stenosis: hemodynamic and clinical improvement after disopyramide. N Engl J Med 1982;307:997–9.

78. Pollick C. Disopyramide in hypertrophic cardiomyopathy, II: noninvasive assessment after oral administration. Am J Cardiol 1988;62:1252–5.

79. Morrow AG, Brockenbrough EC. Surgical treatment of idiopathic hypertrophic subaortic stenosis: technic and hemodynamic results of subaortic ventriculomyotomy. Ann Surg 1961;154:181–9.

80. Morrow AG, Lambrew CT, Braunwald E. Idiopathic hypertrophic subaortic stenosis. II. Operative treatment and the results of pre- and postoperative hemodynamic evaluations. Circulation 1964;30(Suppl 4):120–51.

81. Morrow AG, Reitz BA, Epstein SE, et al. Operative treatment in hypertrophic subaortic stenosis. Techniques, and the results of pre and postoperative assessments in 83 patients. Circulation 1975;52: 88–102.

82. Ommen SR, Maron BJ, Olivotto I, et al. Long-term effects of surgical septal myectomy on survival in patients with obstructive hypertrophic cardiomyopathy. J Am Coll Cardiol 2005;46:470–6.

83. Maron BJ, Roberts WC. The father of septal myectomy for obstructive HCM, who also had HCM. The unbelievable story. J Am Coll Cardiol 2001;67: 2900–3.

84. Said SM, Schaff HV, Abel MD, et al. Transapical approach for apical myectomy and relief of midventricular obstruction in hypertrophic cardiomyopathy. J Card Surg 2012;27:443–8.

85. Nguyen A, Schaff HV, Nishimura RA, et al. Early outcomes of repair of left ventricular apical aneurysms in patients with hypertrophic cardiomyopathy. Circulation 2017;136:1979–81.

86. Schaff HV, Brown ML, Dearani JA, et al. Apical myectomy: a new surgical technique for management of severely symptomatic patients with apical hypertrophic cardiomyopathy. J Thorac Cardiovasc Surg 2010;139:634–40.

87. Sigwart U. Non-surgical myocardial reduction for hypertrophic obstructive cardiomyopathy. Lancet 1995;346:211–4.

88. Veselka J, Jensen MK, Liebregts M, et al. Long-term clinical outcome after alcohol septal ablation for

obstructive hypertrophic cardiomyopathy: results from the Euro-ASA registry. Eur Heart J 2016;37: 1517–23.

89. Zeng Z, Wang F, Dou X, et al. Comparison of percutaneous transluminal septal myocardial ablation versus septal myectomy for the treatment of patients with hypertrophic obstructive cardiomyopathy - a meta analysis. Int J Cardiol 2006;112:80–4.

90. Alam M, Dokainish H, Lakkis NM. Hypertrophic obstructive cardiomyopathy-alcohol septal ablation vs. myectomy: a meta-analysis. Eur Heart J 2009; 30:1080–7.

91. Agarwal S, Tuzcu EM, Desai MY. Updated meta-analysis of septal alcohol ablation versus myectomy for hypertrophic cardiomyopathy. J Am Coll Cardiol 2010;55:823–34.

92. Sorajja P, Pedersen WA, Bae R, et al. First experience with percutaneous mitral valve plication as primary therapy for symptomatic obstructive hypertrophic cardiomyopathy. J Am Coll Cardiol 2016;67:2811–8.

93. Fananapazir L, Cannon RO, Tripodi D, et al. Impact of dual chamber permanent pacing in patients with obstructive hypertrophic cardiomyopathy with symptoms refractory to verapamil and beta-adrenergic blocker therapy. Circulation 1992;85: 2149–61.

94. Fananapazir L, Epstein ND, Curiel RV, et al. Long-term results of dual chamber (DDD) pacing in obstructive hypertrophic cardiomyopathy: evidence for progressive symptomatic and hemodynamic improvement and reduction of left ventricular hypertrophy. Circulation 1994;90: 2731–42.

95. Maron BJ, Nishimura RA, McKenna WJ, et al. Assessment of permanent dual-chamber pacing as a treatment for drug-refractory symptomatic patients with obstructive hypertrophic cardiomyopathy: a randomized, double-blind cross-over study (M-PATHY). Circulation 1999;99:2927–33.

96. Maron BJ, Shen WK, Link MS, et al. Efficacy of implantable cardioverter defibrillators for the prevention of sudden death in patients with hypertrophic cardiomyopathy. N Engl J Med 2000;342: 365–73.

97. O'Mahony C, Jichi F, Pavlou M, et al. A novel clinical risk prediction model for sudden cardiac death in hypertrophic cardiomyopathy (HCM risk-SCD). Eur Heart J 2014;35:2010–20.

98. Ma H, Marti-Gutierrez N, Park SW, et al. Correction of a pathogenic gene mutation in human embryos. Nature 2017;548:413–9.

Echocardiography in the Diagnosis and Management of Hypertrophic Cardiomyopathy

Harry Rakowski, MD, FRCP[a],*, Sarah Hoss, MD[b],
Lynne K. Williams, MBBCh[c]

KEYWORDS

- Cardiomyopathy • Hypertrophy • Echocardiography • Phenotype

KEY POINTS

- Hypertrophic cardiomyopathy is inherited in an autosomal dominant way, but there is often incomplete penetrance and variable phenotype even with the same genotype.
- It is characterized by a degree of hypertrophy, usually asymmetric, that is, not due to another identifiable cause, as well as variable degrees of myocardial fibrosis and microvascular abnormalities.
- Echocardiography has played the greatest single role in assisting clinicians in the diagnosis and management of the complex manifestations of this condition for more than 50 years.

INTRODUCTION

Hypertrophic cardiomyopathy (HCM) is an inherited condition present in about 1/500 individuals with more than 1500 causative mutations identified in primarily 10 sarcomeric proteins. Although HCM is inherited in an autosomal dominant way, there is often incomplete penetrance and variable phenotype even with the same genotype. It is characterized by a degree of hypertrophy (usually asymmetric), that is, not due to another identifiable cause, as well as variable degrees of myocardial fibrosis and microvascular abnormalities. Echocardiography has played the greatest single role in assisting clinicians in the diagnosis and management of the complex manifestations of this condition for more than 50 years. It is essential for the determination of the phenotypic expression of disease, evaluation and management of symptoms arising from dynamic left ventricular outflow tract (LVOT) obstruction, detection of systolic and diastolic dysfunction, and defining prognosis. Recommendations for the use of echocardiography in the evaluation and management of HCM are listed in **Table 1** and its role in the comprehensive assessment of HCM is shown in **Fig. 1**.

DIAGNOSIS OF HYPERTROPHIC CARDIOMYOPATHY AND DETERMINATION OF PHENOTYPE

The clinical diagnosis of HCM depends on the accurate detection and quantitation of the site and extent of abnormal hypertrophy. When septal hypertrophy predominates, the most commonly used cutoff for maximal wall thickness in HCM is 15 mm, with a septal-to-posterior wall ratio of

Disclosure Statement: None.

[a] University of Toronto, Hypertrophic Cardiomyopathy Clinic, Toronto General Hospital, University Health Network, 200 Elizabeth Street, Toronto, Ontario M5G 2C4, Canada; [b] University Health Network, 101 College Street, Toronto, Ontario M5G 1L7, Canada; [c] Papworth Hospital NHS Foundation Trust, Lakeside Cres, Papworth Everard, Cambridge CB23 3RE, UK

* Corresponding author.

E-mail address: Dr.Harry.Rakowski@uhn.ca

Table 1
Recommendations for the use of echocardiography in the evaluation and management of HCM

Transthoracic echocardiography	Initial evaluation for suspected HCM (Class I) Family screening (Class I) HCM patients with a change in clinical status (Class I) After septal ethanol ablation/surgical myectomy (Class I) Routinely every 1–2 y in stable patients (Class IIa)
Exercise echocardiography	Symptomatic patients with no evidence of resting obstruction (Class IIa)
Contrast echocardiography	Suspicion of apical HCM or apical aneurysm (Class IIa) Intraprocedural guidance of septal ethanol ablation (Class I)
Transesophageal echocardiography	Intraoperative guidance of surgical myectomy (Class I)

1.3:1 or greater. In the setting of systemic hypertension, a ratio of septal-to-posterior wall thickness exceeding 1.5:1 is recommended, demonstrating the usually asymmetric nature of the hypertrophy. When family members who may be affected are screened, an unexplained septal thickness of 13 mm may be used to suggest disease presence, particularly when the electrocardiogram (EKG) reading is abnormal. When a pathogenic, disease-causing mutation is detected, particularly in cascade screening, the diagnosis is established; however, the echocardiogram may be normal in early stages of the disease and even minimal hypertrophy may reflect clinical disease onset. The most common mutations are in the myosin heavy chain and myosin-binding protein portions of the cardiac sarcomere. Although it was initially thought that some mutations were associated with either more severe hypertrophy or later disease onset, more recent MRI studies have shown no difference,[1] thus clinical assessment of disease severity by echocardiography and MRI are essential to determine disease severity. Diastolic dysfunction may be the first manifestation of disease onset in some patients. Hypertrophy may develop at any age, but

most commonly develops and progresses during adolescence reflecting the growth of the body. However, some patients develop late-onset disease in their 50s and beyond, and some patients who carry a pathogenic mutation never express clinical disease. Thus serial echocardiographic studies are required to determine the development and progression of hypertrophy, ventricular function, LVOT obstruction, and left atrial (LA) size and function.

Fig. 2 details the most common different patterns and distributions of hypertrophy, including reverse curvature, neutral septum, sigmoid septum, and apical hypertrophy. In addition, infrequently, the greatest hypertrophy may be in the anterolateral wall or the medial portion of the ventricular septum. The degree and location of hypertrophy therefore is quite variable and has significant prognostic implications and thus must be accurately determined. The pattern of hypertrophy is also predictive of the likelihood of a positive genotype as shown. Patients who have reverse curvature or a neutral septum have about a 50% chance of finding a pathogenic mutation, whereas those with focal basal hypertrophy or apical HCM have a yield of less than 20%. Younger patients with HCM patients are more likely to have the reverse curvature morphology compared with the sigmoid septum, which is more commonly seen in HCM of the elderly and may represent a secondary, nonhereditary form of hypertrophy. Patients in the same family may present with different anatomic variants and variable onset and severity of hypertrophy. Other anatomic abnormalities that can be detected include elongation of the mitral leaflets and anterior papillary muscle displacement or direct insertion into a mitral leaflet, which can contribute to LVOT obstruction and mitral regurgitation (MR).

Screening echocardiograms are recommended for first-degree family members of an affected proband usually starting at puberty. If definitive genetic results are not present, follow-up echocardiographic and EKG studies should be repeated every 5 years until at least the age of 50 years or earlier with a change in clinical status. Affected individuals may reasonably have follow-up studies every 1 to 2 years depending on clinical stability.

Cardiac MRI is the only method of quantitating myocardial scar burden and is superior to echocardiography for papillary muscle abnormalities and the presence of myocardial crypts or apical-basal septal muscle bundles that may help identify patients who truly have HCM rather than secondary hypertrophy. MRI is more accurate in the quantitation of wall thickness, particularly when there is an unusual location for the hypertrophy or

Echocardiography in HCM

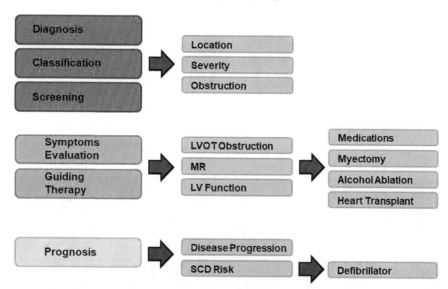

Fig. 1. The role of echocardiography in hypertrophic cardiomyopathy. Echocardiography is a key factor in the diagnosis, assessment, and treatment of patients with HCM. It allows diagnosis of new patients and screening for affected family members, together with classification of the different phenotypes. In symptomatic patients echocardiography is used to evaluate the source of symptoms and assists in choosing the best treatment. It is also a useful tool for sudden cardiac death (SCD) risk stratification by measuring maximal wall thickness, atrial size, and LVOT gradient. It allows us to follow disease progression and the development of heart failure. MR, mitral regurgitation.

predominantly apical involvement. Hindieh and colleagues[2] compared discrepancies between 2-dimensional (2D) echo and MRI measurements of maximal wall thickness and found that in many patients, 2D echo either over- or underestimated the MRI findings. Reasons for discrepancy included focal LV hypertrophy, erroneous inclusion of right ventricular (RV) myocardium, papillary muscles or an apical-basal septal muscle bundle, or an oblique imaging plane. The routine use of myocardial contrast imaging is particularly important when echo image quality is suboptimal. **Fig. 3** demonstrates how contrast-enhanced imaging can better define the septal borders as well as the posterior wall thickness and particularly when lateral wall involvement predominates. In addition, it is often essential to define whether apical HCM is present, to determine the true wall thickness and exclude apically displaced papillary muscles and to define whether an apical aneurysm is present (**Fig. 4**).

LEFT VENTRICULAR OUTFLOW OBSTRUCTION AND MITRAL REGURGITATION

Up to 70% of patients with HCM have dynamic LVOT obstruction, which may be associated with disabling symptoms of dyspnea, chest pain,

presyncope, and syncope. It is also an independent predictor of progression to severe heart failure symptoms, atrial fibrillation (AF), and mortality.[3] In about 30% of patients, obstruction occurs at rest, defined as an LVOT gradient greater than or equal to 30 mm Hg. In about 40% of patients LVOT obstruction occurs with provocation, in response to factors increasing LV contractility, decreasing LV afterload, or reducing LV systolic volume via a reduction in LV preload.[4] **Fig. 5** illustrates the presumed mechanism of LVOT obstruction, which is due to the eject-obstruct-leak concept. Rapid LV ejection occurs through an LVOT narrowed by a hypertrophied basal septum and elongated mitral leaflets that are relatively anteriorly displaced. The resulting Venturi effect and drag forces draw the mitral leaflets toward the septum (systolic anterior motion [SAM]), resulting in leaflet-septal contact, the duration of which reflects the magnitude of the LVOT gradient. The development of SAM also leads to distortion and lack of leaflet coaptation, resulting in MR that is deemed dependent on the obstruction. This MR is typically posteriorly directed due to the funnel created by the SAM and the malcoapting leaflets. Other independent causes of MR should be assessed, such as mitral valve prolapse, torn

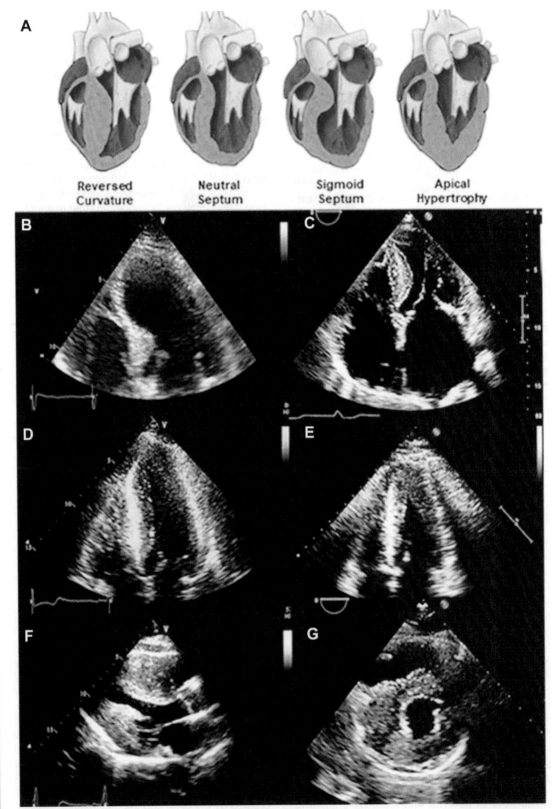

Fig. 2. The different phenotypes of HCM are characterized by the location and extent of hypertrophy. (*A*) Four main phenotypes of HCM. (*B*) Asymmetric septal hypertrophy confined to the basal septum. (*C*) Asymmetric septal

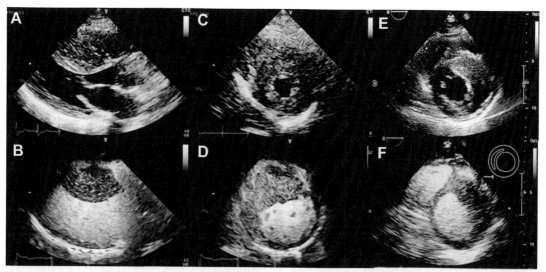

Fig. 3. Using myocardial contrast imaging to accurately define the type of hypertrophy. (*A*) Parasternal long axis view demonstrates septal hypertrophy, but contrast imaging (*B*) reveals massive septal hypertrophy and no significant hypertrophy of the posterior wall. (*C*) What seems like concentric hypertrophy in this short axis view reveals with contrast as asymmetric septal hypertrophy. (*D*) Hypertrophy with unclear wall borders reveals with contrast as anterolateral hypertrophy.

chordae, or mitral annular calcification, which may have a different jet direction (**Fig. 6**). An important clue to non-LVOT obstruction–related MR is that the jet direction is usually central or anteriorly directed rather than the typical posteriorly directed jet. Although the degree of MR can usually be quantitated by 2D echocardiography, 3D imaging is useful when the MR is thought to be independent of the LVOT obstruction, particularly when there is mitral valve prolapse or torn mitral chordae (see **Fig. 6**). The presence of 2 causes of MR namely LVOT obstruction and torn chordae may result in 2 distinct jets of MR with different jet directions.

The LVOT obstruction can be accurately quantitated from continuous wave (CW) Doppler measurements of the LVOT peak velocity (see **Fig. 5**). The Doppler spectral display has a characteristic dagger shape as the gradient starts in early systole with an inflection point around the time of SAM septal contact. This shape of the Doppler profile is useful in distinguishing dynamic from fixed LVOT obstruction, because the onset is earlier than when obstructive gradients occur at the mid-ventricular level (**Fig. 7**) or due to cavity obliteration

gradients that typically occur even later in systole (**Fig. 8**). Another method of distinction is that mid-ventricular obstruction and cavity obliteration should not cause posterior directed MR as is the case with LVOT obstruction and SAM. Contamination of the signal by MR may occur especially when the MR is more central and can be recognized by MR starting earlier in systole, having a larger peak velocity and a different shape. **Fig. 8** demonstrates the ability to unravel 3 different jets that have characteristic shapes that define their origin. The MR jet starts at the onset of systole and is usually more than 6 m per second. The LVOT jet is buried within the combined signals and with a sweep can be unmasked. There is also a third jet, which is late peaking and starts in midsystole and reflects cavity obliteration.

Maximal gradients should be obtained both at rest and following provocation. This can include the use of the Valsalva maneuver, imaging while standing, and most effectively by exercise echocardiography (**Fig. 9**). Outflow gradients are typically treated with beta blockers, verapamil, and/or disopyramide, which reduce the force of LV contraction, and serial echocardiographic studies

hypertrophy with a reverse curvature septum. (*D*) Concentric hypertrophy with a neutral septum. (*E*) Asymmetric apical hypertrophy with hypertrophy confined to the apex. (*F*) Asymmetric massive hypertrophy with diffuse ventricular hypertrophy but extreme hypertrophy of the septum. (*G*) Asymmetric hypertrophy mostly confined to the inferior wall. (*Adapted from* Weissler-Snir A, Crean A, Rakowski H. The role of imaging in the diagnosis and management of hypertrophic cardiomyopathy. Expert Rev Cardiovasc Ther 2016;14(1):52; with permission.)

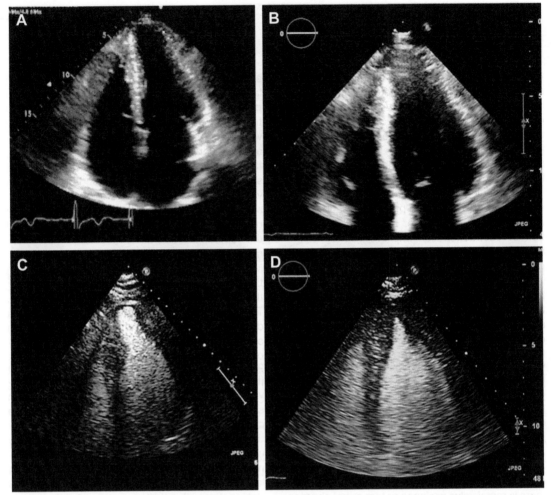

Fig. 4. Accurate echocardiographic imaging of apical HCM with myocardial contrast. (*A, B*) Apical 4-chamber views of 2 patients demonstrate poor definition of the apex. (*C*) Using myocardial contrast reveals one of the patients has apical aneurysm, whereas the other (*D*) presents classic spade-shaped ventricle with no aneurysm. (*Adapted from* Weissler-Snir A, Crean A, Rakowski H. The role of imaging in the diagnosis and management of hypertrophic cardiomyopathy. Expert Rev Cardiovasc Ther 2016;14(1):53; with permission.)

are useful in documenting the response to therapy.

GUIDANCE OF SEPTAL REDUCTION

When medical therapy is not sufficient to adequately relieve moderate or severe obstructive symptoms, invasive septal reduction therapy, either by surgical myectomy or by alcohol septal ablation, should be considered. It is recommended that such procedures be performed in experienced HCM centers with the collaboration of multidisciplinary teams that include expert echocardiography.[5]

Surgical myectomy provides the most immediate and complete relief of LVOT obstruction and can be performed with less than 1% surgical

mortality in experienced centers.[6] Suboptimal myectomy is usually due to removal of inadequate amounts of muscle either in thickness or depth. The key to success is the precise quantitation of the width, length, and circumferential extent of the hypertrophy such that the surgeon can plan to leave only 8 to 10 mm of septal thickness and that the myectomy extends at least 1 cm below the site of septal-leaflet contact (**Fig. 10**). When hypertrophy is more extreme a myectomy may be extended more deeply into the LV with careful avoidance of damage to the papillary muscles. Although myectomy alone is usually sufficient and will alleviate the associated MR, some patients require MV repair or repositioning of the papillary muscle apparatus or have aortic disease requiring valve replacement. Intraoperative TEE

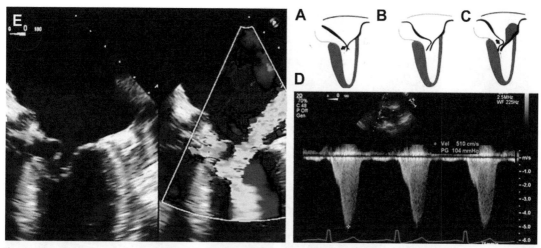

Fig. 5. The mechanism of dynamic LVOT obstruction. (*A*) As systole begins the mitral leaflets, which are often elongated, have a few millimeter of residual leaflet beyond the coaptation point. At early (*B*) and midsystole (*C*), there is anterior and basal movement of the anterior followed by the posterior mitral leaflet (*thick arrow*) with septal contact. This causes malcoaptation of the leaflets and a funnel creating a posterior jet of mitral regurgitation. (*D*) Transesophageal echocardiography imaging of a patient with HCM demonstrates the movement of the anterior mitral leaflet toward the septum causing obstruction and turbulence flow in the LVOT and malcoaptation of the leaflets with posterior jet MR. (*E*) Continuous wave Doppler measurements demonstrate the typical dagger-shaped jet, which can be used to quantitate the LVOT gradient. (*Adapted from* Weissler-Snir A, Crean A, Rakowski H. The role of imaging in the diagnosis and management of hypertrophic cardiomyopathy. Expert Rev Cardiovasc Ther 2016;14(1):55; with permission.)

studies are essential to both plan the surgical approach and to evaluate immediate results postprocedure. Although TEE is the easiest, on occasion when image quality or access is suboptimal, epicardial studies may be useful. Key issues are the successful abolition of the LVOT gradient, lack of persisting midcavity gradients, residual mild or less MR, and avoidance of a ventricular septal defect.

Alcohol septal ablation (ASA) is an important alternative to septal myectomy and is the most frequently performed method of septal reduction in Europe. In North America most patients undergoing ASA are older, have greater comorbidities, and more frequently have focal basal septal hypertrophy. Again significant expertise and a multidisciplinary team are essential to success. One or more septal perforator arteries are usually occluded by ethanol injection. Echocardiography, using contrast perfusion studies, can predict the variable nature of the perfusion bed of the septal perforator artery to be ablated. Its use has greatly improved outcomes by ensuring that an adequate controlled infarct will be obtained and that there is avoidance of infarction of too extensive myocardium or the RV or papillary muscles (**Fig. 11**). The obstructive gradient is typically dramatically reduced in the catheterization laboratory only to increase in the early postprocedure period and

then gradually improve over the next 6 months as the infarcted septum fibroses and shrinks. Myocardial strain studies suggest that the basis for this is the early general myocardial depressant effects of the alcohol injected in all segments, followed by decreased strain only in the infarcted segment.[7]

DIASTOLIC DYSFUNCTION

Diastolic dysfunction is an important feature in all variants of HCM and a significant contributor to symptoms. It likely results from a combination of increased muscle mass, decreased LV volume, increased LV stiffness secondary to myocardial fibrosis, and myocardial disarray and microvascular ischemia. In addition, patients with HCM may have abnormal intracellular calcium and myocardial energetics. Thus there may be impairment in LV relaxation and abnormal diastolic filling with increased LV filling pressures. Although such abnormalities are likely present to some degree in all patients with HCM, it has been difficult to precisely quantitate the degree of abnormality. Initially described echocardiographic findings included reduced mitral E inflow velocity, enhanced A wave velocity, increased duration and velocity of pulmonary A wave reversal, and higher mitral inflow to annular velocity (E/E') ratio. Although

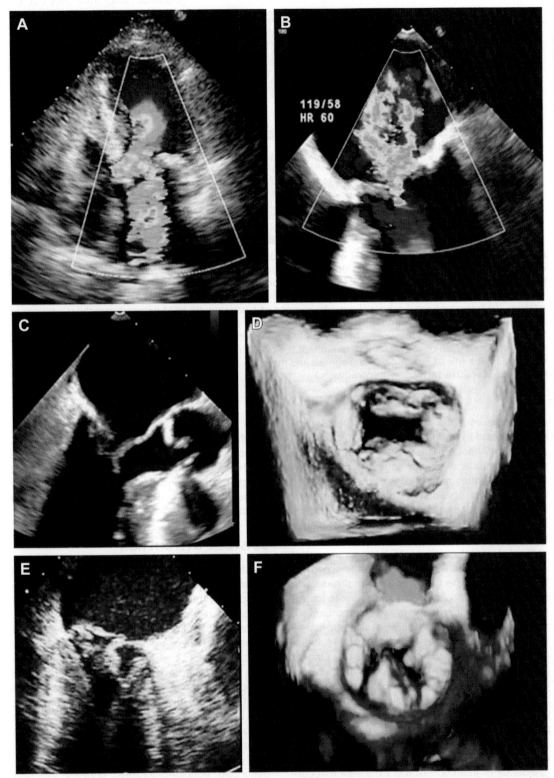

Fig. 6. Assessment of other causes of MR using 2D and 3D echocardiography. (*A–D*) A patient with HCM and MR that is severe with a central jet. Transthoracic echocardiography revealed LVOT turbulent flow (*A*), calcification of the posterior mitral valve leaflet and severe MR with a central jet (*A, B*). (*C*) Transesophageal echocardiography revealed only moderate systolic anterior motion of the anterior mitral leaflet and mitral annular calcification

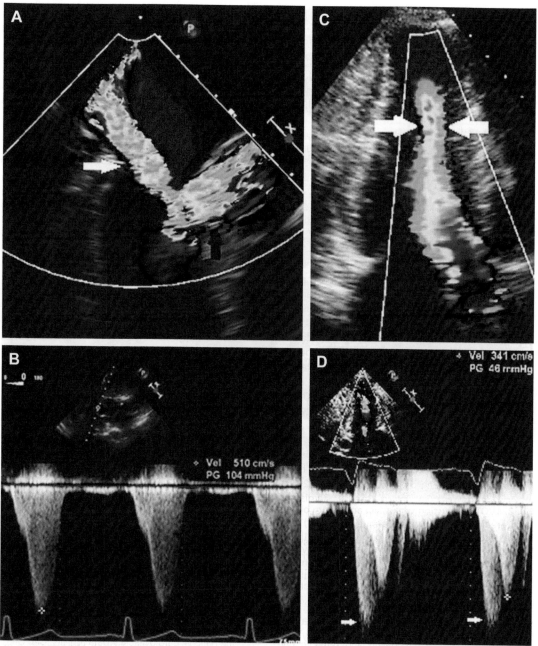

Fig. 7. LVOT versus midventricular obstruction. (*A*) A TEE image with turbulence in the LVOT and associated MR with an eccentric posteriorly directed jet of MR. (*B*) The typical dagger-shaped Doppler signal with a calculated LVOT gradient of 104 mm Hg. (*C*) Mid-cavity obstruction with the turbulent jet in the mid-cavity not the LVOT. (*D*) Two superimposed jets with the left starting with mitral valve closure and due to MR and the right jet starting later and peaking later than the typical LVOT jet and due to mid-cavity obstruction.

extending into the mitral leaflets. Both TEE and 3D echocardiography (*D*) showed that severe MR is mostly due to severe annular and mitral valve calcification. (*E*) TEE presence of both anterior motion of the anterior leaflet with SAM septal contact and a flail posterior mitral leaflet that coapts behind the anterior leaflet. (*F*) A flail P2 segment.

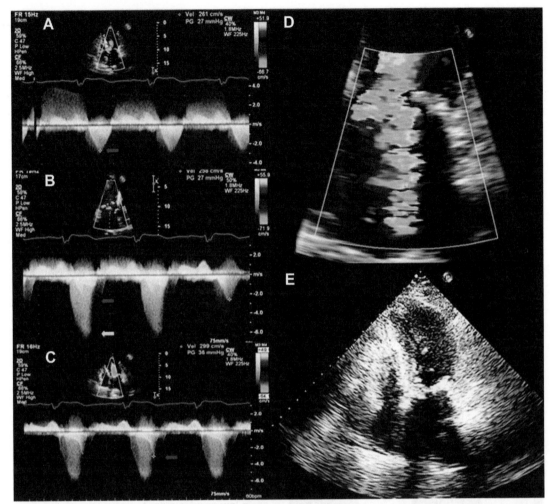

Fig. 8. LVOT obstruction versus MR and cavity obliteration. (*A–C*) Tthe detection of 3 systolic jets. (*A*) A 27-mm LVOT gradient with the typical dagger shape. (*B*) Superimposition with an MR jet of greater than 6 m per second, which starts with mitral valve closure and slightly earlier than the LVOT jet and does not have a dagger shape. With a sweep the jets can be separated as shown in the third beat. (*C*) Superimposition of a cavity obliteration jet, which typically peaks in late systole. (*D*) The mild LVOT obstruction is associated with severe central MR due to mitral annular calcification. (*E*) The severe annular calcification as well as the cavity obliteration.

such measurements are reasonably accurate in patients with abnormal systolic function they lack precision in HCM. Recently the EAE/ASE guidelines recommend using an integrated approach to the assessment of diastolic function by including 4 variables,[8] incorporating the following:

1. Average E/e' ratio greater than 14
2. LA volume index (>34 mL/m^2)
3. Pulmonary vein atrial reversal velocity (Ar-A duration $\geq$ 30 msec)
4. Peak velocity of TR jet by CW Doppler greater than 2.8 m/s

Myocardial mechanics studies may be more sensitive and have demonstrated decreased peak early diastolic to peak systolic strain rate, prolonged time for LV untwisting, and lower apical reverse rotation fraction.[9] Such abnormalities are more common in more symptomatic patients. Despite these advances the precise evaluation of diastolic function remains time consuming and elusive.

LEFT ATRIAL VOLUMES AND FUNCTION

LA volume is often increased in all groups of patients with HCM and reflects abnormalities in myocardial stiffness and the presence of MR due to LVOT obstruction. Although LA size was initially reported, LA volumes indexed to body surface

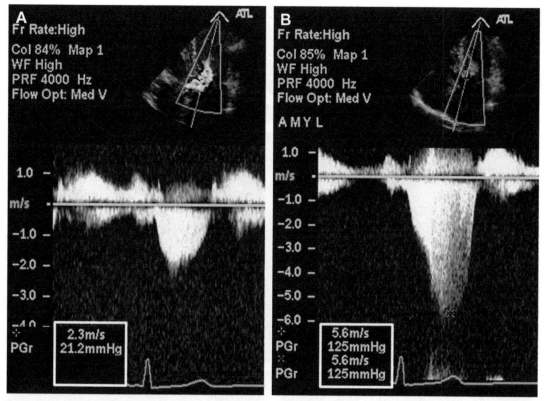

Fig. 9. Provocable LVOT obstruction. (*A*) A resting LVOT gradient of only 21 mm Hg. (*B*) A provocable gradient of 125 mm Hg after the use of amyl nitrite. Note that the Doppler jet has a dagger shape and starts relatively early in systole, demonstrating that it is due to LVOT obstruction and not MR or cavity obliteration. Provocation of gradients can be performed by the use of the Valsalva maneuver, imaging while standing, or, most effectively, by stress echocardiography. (*Adapted from* Weissler-Snir A, Crean A, Rakowski H. The role of imaging in the diagnosis and management of hypertrophic cardiomyopathy. Expert Rev Cardiovasc Ther 2016;14(1):51–74; reprinted by permission of the publisher Taylor & Francis Ltd, http://www.tandfonline.com.)

area provide the greatest reflection of the cumulative effects of LV hypertrophy and stiffness and diastolic function. An LA volume index of greater than 34 mL/m² is associated with a higher risk of development of complications of HCM such as heart failure and AF as well as a higher mortality.[10] Thus measurement of LA volume provides a reliable index of disease severity. In patients with HCM, the LA not only dilates but often has a loss of function. The LA has phasic emptying volumes that reflect both LV filling and atrial function. The LA has an early inflow phase, diastasis, and atrial contraction. Reservoir function represents the enlargement of the LA with storage of pulmonary venous return during ventricular systole and isovolumic relaxation. Conduit function represents the passive emptying of the LA during early relaxation. Booster function is the active emptying of the LA volume into the LV during atrial contraction (**Fig. 12**). Abnormalities of booster pump function have been shown to be a predictor for the development of AF, heart failure, and

hospitalization.[11,12] Other measures of LA function include LA strain and strain rate and LA ejection fraction, which also have prognostic value. Reduction of LVOT obstruction by surgical myectomy has been shown to reduce LA volumes and improve LA function as filling pressures and the degree of MR are reduced.[13]

EVALUATION OF PROGNOSIS AND NATURAL HISTORY
Sudden Cardiac Death

Sudden cardiac death (SCD) is the most feared complication of HCM and is due to ventricular tachyarrhythmias. The incidence of sudden death was initially thought to be about 1% per year, but as more lower-risk patients were included in follow-up assessments the incidence is likely well less than 0.5% per year. Both the AHA-ACC and ESC guidelines list algorithms for the determination of risk of SCD and the use of risk stratification in the recommendations for implantation of

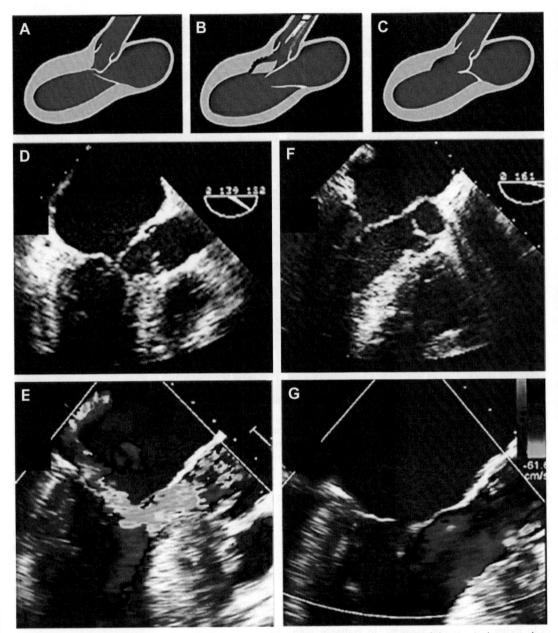

Fig. 10. Intraoperative imaging of surgical myectomy. (*A–C*) A cartoon representation of the surgical approach to myectomy. An aortotomy is made and the aortic leaflets retracted. A section of septal muscle is removed so that there is at least a depth of 1 cm below the site of SAM septal contact. The relatively blind nature of the operative field increases the importance of accurate echo guidance. (*D, E*) The preoperative SAM septal contact with LVOT turbulence and posteriorly directed MR. (*F, G*) Widening of the LVOT following myectomy with resolution of the LVOT turbulence and MR. (*Adapted from* Weissler-Snir A, Crean A, Rakowski H. The role of imaging in the diagnosis and management of hypertrophic cardiomyopathy. Expert Rev Cardiovasc Ther 2016;14(1):51–74; reprinted by permission of the publisher Taylor & Francis Ltd, http://www.tandfonline.com.)

an implantable cardioverter defibrillator (ICD), which may be life-saving. Although these 2 guidelines vary significantly they both incorporate important risk markers detected by echocardiography. The degree of maximal hypertrophy by echocardiography has been shown to be a continuous variable in determining SCD risk and when 30 mm or greater, may alone represent an indication for an ICD. Unexplained syncope is also an important risk factor, and echocardiography is

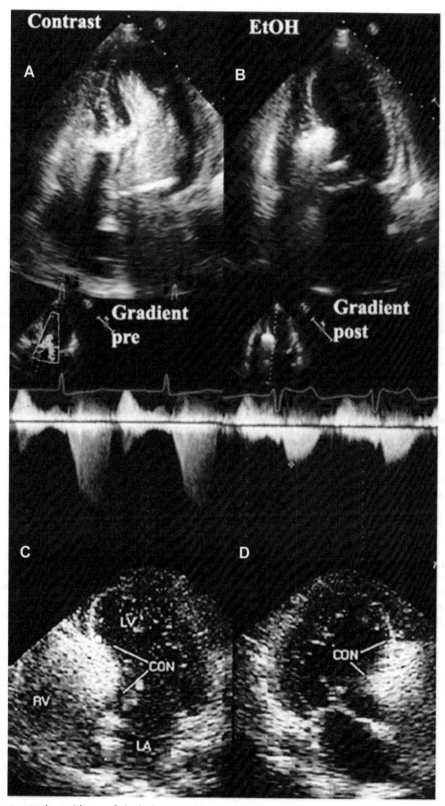

Fig. 11. Contrast echo guidance of alcohol septal ablation. (*A*) Contrast injected into a septal perforator outlining the vascular bed that would be infarcted with alcohol injection. It demonstrates that the territory is appropriate

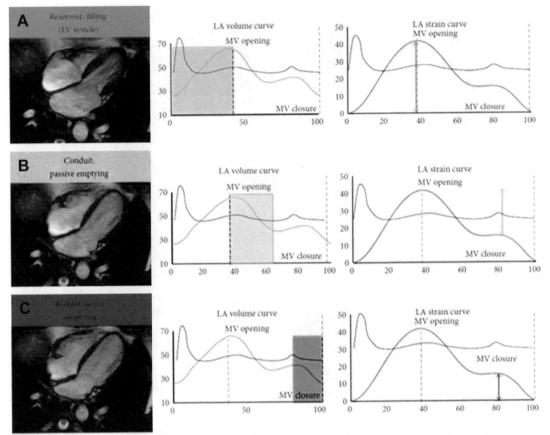

Fig. 12. Stages of LA filling and emptying with associated LA volume and LA strain curves. (*A*) Reservoir filling (*green*) of the LA during LV systole with an increasing LA volume in green and increasing LA strain. (*B*) The conduit phase of passive LA emptying (*yellow*) during early diastole with decreasing LA volume and strain. (*C*) The booster active emptying phase of LA emptying during atrial contraction (*red*) with further decrease in LA volume and strain. (*From* Williams LK, Chan RH, Carasso S, et al. Effect of left ventricular outflow tract obstruction on left atrial mechanics in hypertrophic cardiomyopathy. Biomed Res Int 2015;2015:481245; with permission.)

important to exclude the mechanism of syncope as severe LVOT obstruction, because this represents a modifiable risk factor. Exercise testing, often combined with echocardiography, may show an abnormal blood pressure response to exercise, which may be a useful finding particularly in patients aged 40 years or younger. The ESC guidelines incorporate the severity of LVOT obstruction, as well as LA dimensions, in the risk calculator, whereas the ACC-AHA guidelines do not. Only cardiac MRI studies can determine the degree of myocardial scar, which has more

recently been shown to be an important independent risk factor for SCD. Other important factors in decision-making that can be detected by echocardiography include the presence of apical aneurysms and significant impairment of LV function, as evidenced by an LV ejection fraction of less than 50%.

Heart Failure

Heart failure may occur in the setting of severe LVOT obstruction due to elevated filling pressures

and extends to the level of SAM septal contact. (*B*) The injection of alcohol outlines an infarct bed virtually the same as the contrast bed identified. (*C, D*) The baseline LVOT gradient and the immediate reduction following successful alcohol septal ablation. (*C, D*) Different patient showing a large at-risk septal perfusion bed identified by contrast injection, indicating that this patient is unsuitable for septal alcohol ablation. (*Adapted from* Weissler-Snir A, Crean A, Rakowski H. The role of imaging in the diagnosis and management of hypertrophic cardiomyopathy. Expert Rev Cardiovasc Ther 2016;14(1):51–74; reprinted by permission of the publisher Taylor & Francis Ltd, http://www.tandfonline.com.)

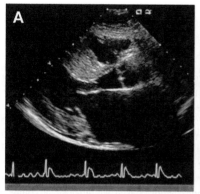
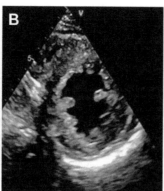
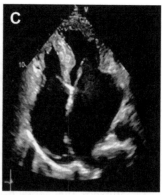

Fig. 13. Progression of LV dysfunction and LA enlargement. (*A*) A study from 2006 from a patient with a 28 mm septum, resting LVOT obstruction, and a normal LV ejection fraction (EF). (*B*) From 2011 shows that the septum is now only 22 mm and the patient had lost his resting LVOT obstruction. (*C*) From 2018 shows that the septum was 21 mm with the development of systolic dysfunction with an EF of 44% and massive LA enlargement. Serial MRI studies showed progressively increasing scar burden as the cause of the loss of systolic function leading to septal thinning and loss of obstruction.

and significant MR. It is usually reversible when due to severe LVOT obstruction that can be effectively managed medically or with septal reduction therapy. As well it may be reversible when due to treated rapid AF. However, up to 10% of patients seen in referral centers may develop heart failure in the absence of LVOT obstruction or rapid AF, and this is usually due to replacement of functioning myocardium by significant scar, severe hypertrophy with diastolic dysfunction or systolic dysfunction, or a combination of both. Such patients may be treated with conventional heart failure medication and if progressive may require advanced therapies such as cardiac resynchronization therapy or as a last resort mechanical circulatory support or cardiac transplantation. **Fig. 13** demonstrates the progression of systolic dysfunction with massive LA enlargement and development of permanent AF.

Echocardiography can assess LV systolic function by the traditional method of calculating ejection fraction; however this does not fully assess LV function. Tissue Doppler studies have shown that decreased lateral mitral annular velocities less than 4 cm/s are associated with occult LV dysfunction, disease progression, and worse prognosis.[14] Myocardial strain studies have also demonstrated a general reduction in longitudinal strain and the magnitude of reduction is also associated with myocardial fibrosis,[15] which is a marker for the development of heart failure and SCD.

DISCRIMINATION OF HYPERTROPHIC CARDIOMYOPATHY FROM PHENOCOPIES

Other conditions may cause initially unexplained hypertrophy and need to be differentiated from HCM because they have different prognosis and management. Differentiation often requires the combined use of echocardiography, genetic testing, and MRI studies. Athlete's heart is benign and is associated with a wall thickness less than 16 mm. The LV cavity is typically larger than with HCM, genetics are negative, hypertrophy regresses with deconditioning, and MRI studies have minimal or no fibrosis. Cardiac amyloidosis is more commonly associated with concentric hypertrophy but may also be asymmetric and even associated with LVOT obstruction in some patients. Distinguishing features may include the presence of RV wall and atrial septal infiltrative thickening, pericardial effusion, and marked biatrial enlargement. Myocardial strain studies usually show apical sparing of longitudinal strain.[16,17] On MRI, late gadolinium enhancement is typically more midwall and diffuse. Anderson Fabry disease also is more likely to have concentric hypertrophy, other systemic abnormalities of the skin, kidneys, eyes, and the peripheral nervous system. Some patients greatly mimic HCM and genetic testing and alpha galactosidase levels can establish the diagnosis.

REFERENCES

1. Weissler-Snir A, Hindieh W, Gruner C, et al. Lack of phenotypic differences by cardiovascular magnetic resonance imaging in MYH7 (beta-Myosin Heavy Chain)- versus MYBPC3 (Myosin-Binding Protein C)-related hypertrophic cardiomyopathy. Circ Cardiovasc Imaging 2017;10 [pii:e005311].
2. Hindieh W, Weissler-Snir A, Hammer H, et al. Discrepant measurements of maximal left ventricular wall thickness between cardiac magnetic resonance

imaging and echocardiography in patients with hypertrophic cardiomyopathy. Circ Cardiovasc Imaging 2017;10 [pii:e006309].

3. Maron MS, Olivotto I, Betocchi S, et al. Effect of left ventricular outflow tract obstruction on clinical outcome in hypertrophic cardiomyopathy. N Engl J Med 2003;348:295–303.

4. Maron MS, Olivotto I, Zenovich AG, et al. Hypertrophic cardiomyopathy is predominantly a disease of left ventricular outflow tract obstruction. Circulation 2006;114:2232–9.

5. Gersh BJ, Maron BJ, Bonow RO, et al, American College of Cardiology Foundation/American Heart Association Task Force on Practice Group. 2011 ACCF/AHA guideline for the diagnosis and treatment of hypertrophic cardiomyopathy: a report of the American College of Cardiology Foundation/ American Heart Association Task Force on Practice Guidelines. Developed in collaboration with the American Association for Thoracic Surgery, American Society of Echocardiography, American Society of Nuclear Cardiology, Heart Failure Society of America, Heart Rhythm Society, Society for Cardiovascular Angiography and Interventions, and Society of Thoracic Surgeons. J Am Coll Cardiol 2011; 58:e212–60.

6. Williams LK, Rakowski H. Surgical myectomy for hypertrophic obstructive cardiomyopathy: the cut that heals. Circulation 2013;128:193–7.

7. Carasso S, Woo A, Yang H, et al. Myocardial mechanics explains the time course of benefit for septal ethanol ablation for hypertrophic cardiomyopathy. J Am Soc Echocardiogr 2008;21:493–9.

8. Cardim N, Galderisi M, Edvardsen T, et al. Role of multimodality cardiac imaging in the management of patients with hypertrophic cardiomyopathy: an expert consensus of the European Association of Cardiovascular Imaging Endorsed by the Saudi Heart Association. Eur Heart J Cardiovasc Imaging 2015;16:280.

9. Carasso S, Yang H, Woo A, et al. Diastolic myocardial mechanics in hypertrophic cardiomyopathy. J Am Soc Echocardiogr 2010;23:164–71.

10. Yang WI, Shim CY, Kim YJ, et al. Left atrial volume index: a predictor of adverse outcome in patients with hypertrophic cardiomyopathy. J Am Soc Echocardiogr 2009;22:1338–43.

11. Rosca M, Popescu BA, Beladan CC, et al. Left atrial dysfunction as a correlate of heart failure symptoms in hypertrophic cardiomyopathy. J Am Soc Echocardiogr 2010;23:1090–8.

12. Paraskevaidis IA, Farmakis D, Papadopoulos C, et al. Two-dimensional strain analysis in patients with hypertrophic cardiomyopathy and normal systolic function: a 12-month follow-up study. Am Heart J 2009;158:444–50.

13. Williams LK, Chan RH, Carasso S, et al. Effect of left ventricular outflow tract obstruction on left atrial mechanics in hypertrophic cardiomyopathy. Biomed Res Int 2015;2015:481245.

14. Bayrak F, Kahveci G, Mutlu B, et al. Tissue Doppler imaging to predict clinical course of patients with hypertrophic cardiomyopathy. Eur J Echocardiogr 2008;9:278–83.

15. Haland TF, Almaas VM, Hasselberg NE, et al. Strain echocardiography is related to fibrosis and ventricular arrhythmias in hypertrophic cardiomyopathy. Eur Heart J Cardiovasc Imaging 2016;17:613–21.

16. Williams LK, Forero JF, Popovic ZB, et al. Patterns of CMR measured longitudinal strain and its association with late gadolinium enhancement in patients with cardiac amyloidosis and its mimics. J Cardiovasc Magn Reson 2017;19:61.

17. Phelan D, Collier P, Thavendiranathan P, et al. Relative apical sparing of longitudinal strain using two-dimensional speckle-tracking echocardiography is both sensitive and specific for the diagnosis of cardiac amyloidosis. Heart 2012;98:1442–8.

Cardiac Magnetic Resonance for Diagnosis and Risk Stratification

Abdallah Sanaani, MD[a], Anthon Fuisz, MD[b],*

KEYWORDS

- Cardiac MRI • Hypertrophic cardiomyopathy • Imaging

KEY POINTS

- Cardiac MRI (CMR) is used in the diagnosis of patients with hypertrophic cardiomyopathy (HCM) through accurate measurements of wall thickness, myocardial mass, and morphologic features.
- CMR is used in assessing the prognosis of patients with HCM through the detection of fibrosis and infarction.
- CMR is useful in distinguishing HCM from other similar-appearing disease entities.

INTRODUCTION

Cardiac MRI (CMR) has several unique features that are useful in the care of patients with hypertrophic cardiomyopathy (HCM). The ability to accurately measure left ventricular (LV) wall thickness, LV mass, and ejection fraction as well as quantify mitral regurgitation (MR) that might result from high outflow tract velocities is unique. Add to this the novel aspects of CMR, the ability to detect and measure macroscopic fibrosis through late gadolinium enhancement (LGE), myocardial perfusion, and more subtle alterations in myocardial fibrosis through T1 mapping, and CMR becomes indispensable for the initial evaluation and long-term care of patients with HCM (**Figs. 1** and **2**). Furthermore, prognostic information regarding the risk of sudden cardiac death (SCD) and risk of heart failure can be derived from the CMR data points, adding to the usefulness for the clinician.

The standard CMR examination in the presumed HCM patient should include cine sequences to allow for ejection fraction, wall thickness, and myocardial mass to be determined. Views of the outflow tract likewise should be performed to demonstrate turbulence and the interaction with the mitral valve apparatus. Flow measures in the aorta are helpful to allow the quantification of MR should it occur. If there is any remaining concern for aortic stenosis, cine views of the aortic valve can be performed. T1 mapping sequences should be done as well as the standard post–gadolinium scar imaging. Resting myocardial perfusion imaging may also provide helpful data. Postprocessing should include the calculation of LV mass, and the percent scar, if fibrosis is detected.

MORPHOLOGY AND MEASUREMENTS
Wall Thickness

Accurate LV wall thickness measurement is an integral component in the initial diagnosis of HCM. Generally, for adults, a wall thickness of 15 mm or more is accepted as the cutoff value; this is especially true when the wall thickness is asymmetric.[1,2] Maximum LV wall thickness is a significant predictor of SCD, and a maximum wall thickness of more than 30 mm is the cutoff, as

Disclosure: None.
[a] Gunderson Health System, La Crosse Campus, 1900 South Avenue, La Crosse, WI 54601, USA; [b] Westchester Medical Center, 100 Woods Road, Macy 132, Valhalla, NY 10595, USA
* Corresponding author.
E-mail address: anthon.fuisz@wmchealth.org

Cardiol Clin 37 (2019) 27–33
https://doi.org/10.1016/j.ccl.2018.08.002
0733-8651/19/© 2018 Elsevier Inc. All rights reserved.

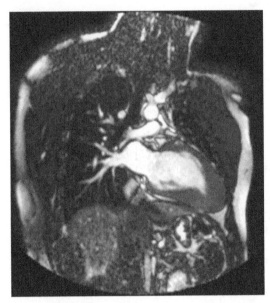

Fig. 1. Apical HCM.

such accurate measurements of the LV wall thickness have implications on management decision in addition to the initial diagnosis.[1,2]

CMR imaging through different anatomic and functional sequences produces definitions of the LV walls with high spatial resolution; the images can be performed through any chosen planes with the same resolution throughout the image. This is in contrast to transthoracic echocardiogram (TTE) in which the spatial resolution is diminished with depth (structures further from the

imaging probe are more challenging to image clearly). CMR images are highly reproducible and are not affected by the body habitus that usually affects ultrasound imaging and leads to suboptimal acoustic windows. Balanced steady-state free precession (bSSFP) is typically the sequence used to assess the morphology function and perform the measurements. CMR measurements are obtained typically from a cine bSSFP sequence at end diastole: either in the basal short axis slice or in the 3-chamber view; immediately basal to the tips of the papillary muscles.[3] The maximum wall thickness is obtained from the short-axis slice stacks measuring the thickest portion of the wall.

CMR was demonstrated to have better reproducibility and interobserver variability of wall thickness measurements than TTE. It is especially useful for the measurement of the inferolateral wall (furthest from the TTE probe) and in patients with suboptimal acoustic windows. Maximum wall thickness measured by CMR tends to be smaller than the TTE measurements. In one small study, CMR maximum wall thickness better correlated with measurements obtained by contrast TTE. The overestimation on some TTE measurements may result from the inclusion of the right ventricular (RV) myocardium, LV trabeculation, papillary muscles, or apical septal bundle.[4–8] The implications of this discrepancy remain to be defined, because the currently used predictors were derived from TTE studies. One study comparing maximal LV wall thickness between CMR and TTE reported that 49.7% of patients were identified to have intermodal measurement discrepancies ≥10%. In 15.9% of patients, measurement discrepancy occurred at diagnostic or prognostic cutoffs.[7]

Left Ventricular Mass

LV mass can be accurately measured by CMR and is free of geometric assumptions. However, this parameter has no utility in the diagnosis, because it has been demonstrated that a significant proportion of patients with a definitive diagnosis of HCM have normal LV mass. Furthermore, it correlates poorly with the maximal wall thickness. However, it might have a prognostic value; markedly increased LV mass index proved more sensitive in predicting outcome than maximal wall thickness but with poor specificity.[9]

MORPHOLOGY AND HYPERTROPHIC CARDIOMYOPATHY VARIANTS

CMR is helpful in differentiating HCM morphology variants and defining the exact distribution of the

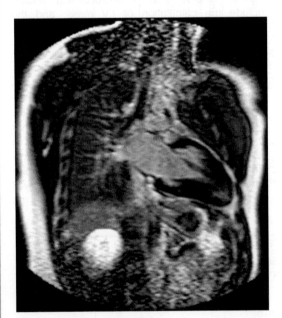

Fig. 2. Fibrosis in apical HCM.

myocardial hypertrophy. It is particularly useful in the apical hypertrophy variant and in sorting out midcavity obstruction with an apical aneurysm from proper apical hypertrophy. It is also helpful in demonstrating hypertrophy affecting the RV wall. These variants are usually difficult to define by TTE and can be misdiagnosed or mistyped. Accurate typing is essential because different variants carry different prognosis and clinical course.[10–13]

LEFT VENTRICULAR OUTFLOW TRACT OBSTRUCTION AND MITRAL REGURGITATION

Dynamic left ventricular outflow tract (LVOT) obstruction due to systolic anterior motion (SAM) of the mitral valve is one of the critical features of obstructive HCM; its severity strongly correlates with the symptoms and prognosis and guides the need for intervention.[14] The LVOT gradient can be measured by a phase velocity CMR sequence; however, it is more reliable and better served by TTE given its dynamic nature. However, CMR has a vital role in determining the mechanism of the LVOT obstruction. Dynamic LVOT obstruction in HCM is typically caused by the SAM of the anterior mitral valve leaflet toward the thick basal septum. The subvalvular apparatus (displaced chordae/papillary muscle) and posterior mitral valve leaflets can contribute to the phenomena as well. Through its high spatial and temporal resolution, CMR can visualize the degree to which different components (mitral valve leaflets, displaced chordae/papillary muscles, and thickened septum) contribute to the obstruction. This interaction has different patterns and should be determined for each patient to plan and tailor the most appropriate intervention.[15–19] CMR is also useful in determining the mechanism and degree of the associated MR; regurgitant volume and fraction can be measured by comparing the LV stroke volume to the forward flow measured directly in the ascending aorta. This method has excellent accuracy and reproducibility and is considered the gold standard to determine the MR degree.[19–21] CMR is also useful to exclude other associated anomalies of the aortic valve and the aorta (bicuspid aortic valve, aortic stenosis, aortic regurgitation, coarctation, and aortic aneurysm), especially before a planned intervention. Last, CMR can be used to localize the infarction created in catheter-based septal remodeling.

LATE GADOLINIUM ENHANCEMENT

LGE is based on the kinetic behavior of gadolinium that washes out slower from diseased myocardium, due to fibrosis, infarction, or myocyte necrosis, compared with the healthy myocardium (**Fig. 3**). It is established as a reliable method able to accurately delineate the extent of fibrosis compared with a histologic specimen in nonischemic and ischemic cardiomyopathy alike. In HCM, the pattern of LGE is usually a focal area of midmyocardial fibrosis localized to the site of maximum wall thickness as well as at the RV insertion points.[12,22–24] The extent of fibrosis on LGE correlated with the severity of the phenotype, onset of heart failure, mortality, and poorer outcomes.[12,25–28] Recently, more interest has been focused on its ability to predict SCD; numerous studies have reported an association between the extent of LGE and the onset of NSVT, VT, and SCD in HCM.[29–32] Automated postprocessing analysis for the quantification of the percentage of DHE is available through different vendors. An important recent study demonstrated that with the presence of LGE of $\geq$20% of LV myocardium identified patients at higher risk for major adverse cardiac arrhythmic events, even in the absence of other conventional predictors of SCD. In contrast, LGE less than 20% was associated with a lower risk of major adverse cardiac arrhythmic events, even in the presence of traditional predictors of SCD.[33]

NATIVE T1 AND T1 MAPPING

Each tissue, including healthy myocardium, has a specific T1 relaxation time. Alteration of the healthy myocardium by extracellular deposition, including fibrosis, alters its magnetic properties, leading to prolongation of the T1 relaxation time.

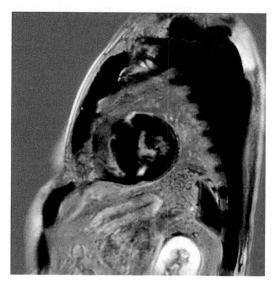

Fig. 3. Fibrosis in HCM.

The degree to which T1 time is prolonged correlates with the degree of extracellular deposition. T1 mapping is obtained by measuring the T1 time throughout a myocardial slice; this allows measuring an average T1 time value as well as a value for each segment. The extracellular deposition is different depending on the disease process. In HCM, native T1 has been proposed as a noncontrast measure of fibrosis. Native T1 time is most prolonged in areas of LGE but is also abnormally prolonged to a lesser degree in areas free from DHE, making it a potential earlier marker of fibrosis. Averaged prolonged T1 time has been linked in histologic studies to diffuse fibrosis.[34–36] It is also useful to differentiate HCM from other cause of hypertrophy as discussed later in a separate section.[37,38] Prolonged native T1 time in cardiomyopathy, in general, is associated with poorer outcomes (mortality, cardiovascular mortality, and heart failure).[39,40] However, large-scale studies looking at outcomes specific to HCM or SCD in HCM are lacking. T1 values themselves are vendor and sequence dependent however, so the utilization of this finding requires local CMR laboratories to develop normal ranges for patients or phantom-derived values to be fully implemented.

MYOCARDIAL PERFUSION

Perfusion imaging has been shown to be of value as well in HCM patients. Resting perfusion abnormalities correlate to areas of fibrosis and to maximal wall thickness. When these areas are found to coexist with areas of fibrosis, they are associated with an increased incidence of nonsustained ventricular tachycardia.[41] New techniques that allow quantitative myocardial perfusion on the pixel level have also identified abnormalities in appropriate hyperemic myocardial blood flow in areas of fibrosis in some patients with HCM.[42]

OTHER DISEASE ENTITIES

Another advantage of CMR is the ability to distinguish HCM from other entities that share the common feature of thickened LV walls. Other than the accurate measurement of wall thickness, it is the CMR techniques that allow tissue characterization that are the most useful. Although there still can be some overlap, these techniques can provide another piece of data to add to existing clinical history.

Distinguishing between hypertrophy due to hypertension (HTN) or to HCM can be clinically difficult. The observation of higher T1 values in HCM compared with those observed in HTN can be helpful in making this delineation. This difference also exists in the patient carrying an HCM gene but not yet manifesting the phenotype.[37]

Distinguishing the athlete's heart and the adaptation that can occur in certain sports is another area of overlap with HCM, especially in the gray zone of only slightly abnormal wall thickness. The presence of delayed hyperenhancement as a marker of fibrosis can help establish the diagnosis of HCM, as can accurate wall measurements if a patient is removed from the activity with the intention of allowing the heart to return to normal.[43]

Fabry disease is often first recognized by marked hypertrophy noted with echocardiography. By CMR techniques, Fabry disease can be distinguished by midwall delayed hyperenhancement, classically crescent-shaped, and seen in the lateral wall, as well as by lower than normal T1 values.

Cardiac amyloid is another entity associated with thick ventricular walls. The diffuse pattern of enhancement after gadolinium injection is the most helpful feature to distinguish the patient with amyloid from the one with HCM. T1 values are likewise higher in amyloid.

Last, the patient with a cardiac tumor may present with segmental apparent hypertrophy of myocardial segments. Cardiac lymphoma (**Fig. 4**) and cardiac fibroma are 2 examples. In most cases, different T1 and T2 appearance and differential response to gadolinium, both on initial perfusion and in delayed images, will allow for these patients to be identified and HCM excluded.

The ability of CMR to provide accurate measurements and unique insights into the tissue characteristics of the hypertrophic heart makes it a very useful technique for establishing both the diagnosis and the prognosis. Similarly, these strengths can be used to separate the HCM patient from other entities that might otherwise appear similar

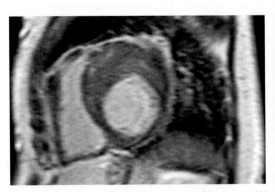

Fig. 4. Cardiac lymphoma appearing as LV hypertrophy.

by different imaging techniques. Adding in the ability to measure regurgitation and perfusion abnormalities and CMR becomes the "one-stop shop" for HCM.

REFERENCES

1. Gersh BJ, Maron BJ, Bonow RO, et al. 2011 ACCF/AHA guideline for the diagnosis and treatment of hypertrophic cardiomyopathy. J Am Coll Cardiol 2011;58(25):e212–60. Available at: http://linkinghub.elsevier.com/retrieve/pii/S0735109711022753. Accessed April 27, 2018.

2. Elliott PM, Anastasakis A, Borger MA, et al. 2014 ESC Guidelines on diagnosis and management of hypertrophic cardiomyopathy. Eur Heart J 2014;35(39):2733–79. Available at: https://academic.oup.com/eurheartj/article-lookup/doi/10.1093/eurheartj/ehu284. Accessed April 27, 2018.

3. Schulz-Menger J, Bluemke DA, Bremerich J, et al. Standardized image interpretation and post processing in cardiovascular magnetic resonance: society for cardiovascular magnetic resonance (SCMR) board of trustees task force on standardized post processing. J Cardiovasc Magn Reson 2013;15(1):35. Available at: http://jcmr-online.biomedcentral.com/articles/10.1186/1532-429X-15-35. Accessed April 28, 2018.

4. Devlin AM, Moore NR, Ostman-Smith I. A comparison of MRI and echocardiography in hypertrophic cardiomyopathy. Br J Radiol 1999;72(855):258–64. Available at: http://www.ncbi.nlm.nih.gov/pubmed/10396215. Accessed April 28, 2018.

5. Bois JP, Geske JB, Foley TA, et al. Comparison of maximal wall thickness in hypertrophic cardiomyopathy differs between magnetic resonance imaging and transthoracic echocardiography. Am J Cardiol 2017;119(4):643–50. Available at: http://www.ncbi.nlm.nih.gov/pubmed/27956002. Accessed April 28, 2018.

6. Corona-Villalobos CP, Sorensen LL, Pozios I, et al. Left ventricular wall thickness in patients with hypertrophic cardiomyopathy: a comparison between cardiac magnetic resonance imaging and echocardiography. Int J Cardiovasc Imaging 2016;32(6):945–54. Available at: http://www.ncbi.nlm.nih.gov/pubmed/26896038. Accessed April 27, 2018.

7. Hindieh W, Weissler-Snir A, Hammer H, et al. Discrepant measurements of maximal left ventricular wall thickness between cardiac magnetic resonance imaging and echocardiography in patients with hypertrophic cardiomyopathyclinical perspective. Circ Cardiovasc Imaging 2017;10(8):e006309. Available at: http://circimaging.ahajournals.org/lookup/doi/10.1161/CIRCIMAGING.117.006309. Accessed April 27, 2018.

8. Webb J, Villa A, Bekri I, et al. Usefulness of cardiac magnetic resonance imaging to measure left ventricular wall thickness for determining risk scores for sudden cardiac death in patients with hypertrophic cardiomyopathy. Am J Cardiol 2017;119(9):1450–5. Available at: http://www.ncbi.nlm.nih.gov/pubmed/28267963. Accessed April 28, 2018.

9. Olivotto I, Maron M, Autore C, et al. Assessment and significance of left ventricular mass by cardiovascular magnetic resonance in hypertrophic cardiomyopathy. Elsevier; 2008. Available at: https://www.sciencedirect.com/science/article/pii/S0735109708018640. Accessed April 27, 2018.

10. Harada K, Shimizu T, Sugishita Y, et al. Hypertrophic cardiomyopathy with midventricular obstruction and apical aneurysm: a case report. Jpn Circ J 2001;65(10):915–9. Available at: http://www.ncbi.nlm.nih.gov/pubmed/11665799. Accessed April 28, 2018.

11. Ibrahim T, Schwaiger M. Diagnosis of apical hypertrophic cardiomyopathy using magnetic resonance imaging. Heart 2000;83(1):E1. Available at: http://www.ncbi.nlm.nih.gov/pubmed/10618355. Accessed April 28, 2018.

12. Moon JCC, Fisher NG, McKenna WJ, et al. Detection of apical hypertrophic cardiomyopathy by cardiovascular magnetic resonance in patients with non-diagnostic echocardiography. Heart 2004;90(6):645–9. Available at: http://www.ncbi.nlm.nih.gov/pubmed/15145868. Accessed April 28, 2018.

13. Maron MS, Hauser TH, Dubrow E, et al. Right ventricular involvement in hypertrophic cardiomyopathy. Am J Cardiol 2007;100(8):1293–8. Available at: http://www.ncbi.nlm.nih.gov/pubmed/17920373. Accessed April 28, 2018.

14. Autore C, Bernabò P, Stella Barillà C, et al. The prognostic importance of left ventricular outflow obstruction in hypertrophic cardiomyopathy varies in relation to the severity of symptoms. J Am Coll Cardiol 2005;45(7):1076–80. Accessed August 8, 2018.

15. Harrigan CJ, Appelbaum E, Maron BJ, et al. Significance of papillary muscle abnormalities identified by cardiovascular magnetic resonance in hypertrophic cardiomyopathy. Am J Cardiol 2008;101(5):668–73. Available at: http://www.ncbi.nlm.nih.gov/pubmed/18308018. Accessed April 28, 2018.

16. Klues HG, Roberts WC, Maron BJ. Anomalous insertion of papillary muscle directly into anterior mitral leaflet in hypertrophic cardiomyopathy. Significance in producing left ventricular outflow obstruction. Circulation 1991;84(3):1188–97. Available at: http://www.ncbi.nlm.nih.gov/pubmed/1884449. Accessed April 28, 2018.

17. Kon MW, Grech ED, Ho SY, et al. Anomalous papillary muscle as a cause of left ventricular outflow tract obstruction in an adult. Ann Thorac Surg 1997;63(1):232–4. Available at: http://www.ncbi.nlm.nih.gov/pubmed/8993276. Accessed April 28, 2018.

18. Maron MS, Olivotto I, Harrigan C, et al. Mitral Valve abnormalities identified by cardiovascular magnetic resonance represent a primary phenotypic expression of hypertrophic cardiomyopathy. Circulation 2011;124(1):40–7. Available at: http://www.ncbi.nlm.nih.gov/pubmed/21670234. Accessed April 28, 2018.

19. Patel P, Dhillon A, Popovic ZB, et al. Left ventricular outflow tract obstruction in hypertrophic cardiomyopathy patients without severe septal hypertrophy: implications of mitral valve and papillary muscle abnormalities assessed using cardiac magnetic resonance and echocardiography. Circ Cardiovasc Imaging 2015;8(7):e003132. Available at: http://www.ncbi.nlm.nih.gov/pubmed/26082555. Accessed April 28, 2018.

20. Uretsky S, Gillam L, Lang R, et al. Discordance between echocardiography and MRI in the assessment of mitral regurgitation severity. J Am Coll Cardiol 2015;65(11):1078–88. Available at: http://www.ncbi.nlm.nih.gov/pubmed/25790878. Accessed April 28, 2018.

21. Penicka M, Vecera J, Mirica DC, et al. Prognostic implications of magnetic resonance-derived quantification in asymptomatic patients with organic mitral regurgitation: comparison with Doppler echocardiography-derived integrative approach. Circulation 2018;137(13):1349–60. Available at: http://www.ncbi.nlm.nih.gov/pubmed/29269390. Accessed April 28, 2018.

22. Vermes E, Carbone I, Friedrich MG, et al. Patterns of myocardial late enhancement: typical and atypical features. Arch Cardiovasc Dis 2012;105(5):300–8. Available at: https://www.sciencedirect.com/science/article/pii/S1875213612000332#bib0065. Accessed April 29, 2018.

23. Satoh H, Sano M, Suwa K, et al. Distribution of late gadolinium enhancement in various types of cardiomyopathies: significance in differential diagnosis, clinical features and prognosis. World J Cardiol 2014;6(7):585–601. Available at: http://www.ncbi.nlm.nih.gov/pubmed/25068019. Accessed April 29, 2018.

24. Teraoka K, Hirano M, Ookubo H, et al. Delayed contrast enhancement of MRI in hypertrophic cardiomyopathy. Magn Reson Imaging 2004;22(2):155–61. Available at: http://www.ncbi.nlm.nih.gov/pubmed/15010107. Accessed April 29, 2018.

25. Briasoulis A, Mallikethi-Reddy S, Palla M, et al. Myocardial fibrosis on cardiac magnetic resonance and cardiac outcomes in hypertrophic cardiomyopathy: a meta-analysis. Heart 2015;101(17):1406–11.

26. Hanna C, Lesser JR, Udelson JE, et al. Clinical profile and significance of delayed enhancement in hypertrophic cardiomyopathy. Circ Heart Fail 2008;1:184–91. Available at: http://circheartfailure.

ahajournals.org/content/1/3/184.full. Accessed April 29, 2018.

27. Klopotowski M, Kukula K, Malek LA, et al. The value of cardiac magnetic resonance and distribution of late gadolinium enhancement for risk stratification of sudden cardiac death in patients with hypertrophic cardiomyopathy. J Cardiol 2016;68(1):49–56.

28. O'Hanlon R, Grasso A, Roughton M, et al. Prognostic significance of myocardial fibrosis in hypertrophic cardiomyopathy. J Am Coll Cardiol 2010;56(11):867–74. Available at: https://www.sciencedirect.com/science/article/pii/S0735109710019169. Accessed April 29, 2018.

29. Chan RH, Maron BJ, Olivotto I, et al. Prognostic value of quantitative contrast-enhanced cardiovascular magnetic resonance for the evaluation of sudden death risk in patients with hypertrophic cardiomyopathy. Circulation 2014;130(6):484–95.

30. Fluechter S, Kuschyk J, Wolpert C, et al. Extent of late gadolinium enhancement detected by cardiovascular magnetic resonance correlates with the inducibility of ventricular tachyarrhythmia in hypertrophic cardiomyopathy. J Cardiovasc Magn Reson 2010;12:30.

31. Suk T, Edwards C, Hart H, et al. Myocardial scar detected by contrast-enhanced cardiac magnetic resonance imaging is associated with ventricular tachycardia in hypertrophic cardiomyopathy patients. Heart Lung Circ 2008;17(5):370–4.

32. Weng Z, Yao J, Chan RH, et al. Prognostic value of LGE-CMR in HCM: a meta-analysis. JACC Cardiovasc Imaging 2016;9(12):1392–402.

33. Doesch C, Tülümen E, Akin I, et al. Incremental benefit of late gadolinium cardiac magnetic resonance imaging for risk stratification in patients with hypertrophic cardiomyopathy. Sci Rep 2017;7(1):6336. Available at: http://www.nature.com/articles/s41598-017-06533-0. Accessed April 29, 2018.

34. Dass S, Suttie JJ, Piechnik SK, et al. Myocardial tissue characterization using magnetic resonance noncontrast T1 mapping in hypertrophic and dilated cardiomyopathy. Circ Cardiovasc Imaging 2012;5(6):726–33.

35. Iles LM, Ellims AH, Llewellyn H, et al. Histological validation of cardiac magnetic resonance analysis of regional and diffuse interstitial myocardial fibrosis. Eur Heart J Cardiovasc Imaging 2015;16(1):14–22.

36. Małek ŁA, Werys K, Kłopotowski M, et al. Native T1-mapping for non-contrast assessment of myocardial fibrosis in patients with hypertrophic cardiomyopathy - comparison with late enhancement quantification. Magn Reson Imaging 2015;33(6):718–24.

37. Hinojar R, Varma N, Child N, et al. T1 mapping in discrimination of hypertrophic phenotypes: hypertensive heart disease and hypertrophic cardiomyopathy: findings from the international T1 multicenter

cardiovascular magnetic resonance study. Circ Cardiovasc Imaging 2015;8(12) [pii:e003285].

38. Puntmann VO, Voigt T, Chen Z, et al. Native T1 mapping in differentiation of normal myocardium from diffuse disease in hypertrophic and dilated cardiomyopathy. JACC Cardiovasc Imaging 2013;6(4):475–84. Available at: https://www.sciencedirect.com/science/article/pii/S1936878X13001344. Accessed April 29, 2018.

39. Puntmann VO, Carr-White G, Jabbour A, et al. T1-Mapping and outcome in nonischemic cardiomyopathy. JACC Cardiovasc Imaging 2016;9(1): 40–50. Available at: http://www.ncbi.nlm.nih.gov/pubmed/26762873. Accessed April 30, 2018.

40. Puntmann VO, Carr-White G, Jabbour A, et al. Native T1 and ECV of noninfarcted myocardium and outcome in patients with coronary artery disease.

J Am Coll Cardiol 2018;71(7):766–78. Available at: http://www.ncbi.nlm.nih.gov/pubmed/29447739. Accessed April 30, 2018.

41. Chiribiri A, Leuzzi S, Conte MR, et al. Rest perfusion abnormalities in hypertrophic cardiomyopathy: correlation with myocardial fibrosis and risk factors for sudden cardiac death. Clin Radiol 2015;70(5): 495–501.

42. Ismail TF, Hsu LY, Greve AM, et al. Coronary microvascular ischemia in hypertrophic cardiomyopathy - a pixel-wise quantitative cardiovascular magnetic resonance perfusion study. J Cardiovasc Magn Reson 2014;16:49.

43. Mousavi N, Czarnecki A, Kumar K, et al. Relation of biomarkers and cardiac magnetic resonance imaging after marathon running. Am J Cardiol 2009; 103:1467–72.

Genetic Testing and Counseling for Hypertrophic Cardiomyopathy

Allison L. Cirino, MS[a], Christine E. Seidman, MD[a,b,c],
Carolyn Y. Ho, MD[a,*]

KEYWORDS

• Genetic testing • Genetic counseling • Hypertrophic cardiomyopathy • Pedigree

KEY POINTS

- Hypertrophic cardiomyopathy (HCM) is an autosomal dominant condition caused by DNA variants in genes encoding sarcomere proteins.
- Genetic testing can provide valuable information for patients and families, and it should be considered in the management of patients with HCM.
- Pretest and posttest genetic counseling enables fully informed consent, establishes appropriate expectations, and supports patient adjustment to and understanding of results.
- For families to realize the potential benefit of HCM genetic testing, providers must facilitate information sharing within the family.
- Genetic testing should be coordinated by providers with the requisite expertise to properly interpret results; this may involve collaboration with or referral to specialized providers.

INTRODUCTION

Hypertrophic cardiomyopathy (HCM) is often genetic and most frequently caused by mutations in genes encoding the cardiac sarcomere, the contractile unit of the cardiomyocyte. It is one of the most common inherited cardiovascular conditions. As such, caring for patients with HCM also requires caring for their families. HCM is an autosomal dominant condition, meaning first-degree relatives (parents, siblings, and children) each have a 50% chance of inheriting the genetic variant that causes disease. Guidelines suggest longitudinal screening with echocardiogram and electrocardiogram for first-degree relatives.[1–3] The frequency of evaluation is based on age given the age-dependent penetrance of phenotypic features of HCM. Family screening serves to identify relatives with previously unrecognized HCM and to monitor unaffected relatives for disease development.[4]

Over the past decade, genetic testing has moved beyond the setting of the research laboratory and is routinely offered in HCM clinics to identify the genetic cause of disease in a patient, an approach supported by various professional guidelines.[1–3] Knowledge of the precise genetic cause of disease can improve diagnostic accuracy in a patient, thus refining their care, and can improve family management by identifying relatives with unrecognized HCM or at risk for developing HCM, as well as relatives who do not need

Disclosure Statement: C.Y. Ho receives research support from MyoKardia, Inc. C.E. Seidman is a founder of MyoKardia. C.Y. Ho and A.L. Cirino are supported by funding from the National Institutes of Health (1P50HL112349 to C.Y. Ho).

[a] Cardiovascular Division, Brigham and Women's Hospital, 75 Francis Street, Boston, MA 02115, USA; [b] Department of Genetics, Harvard Medical School, NRB 256, 77 Avenue Louis Pasteur, Boston, MA 02115, USA; [c] Howard Hughes Medical Institute, HHMI Investigator Program, 4000 Jones Bridge Road, Chevy Chase, MD 20815, USA
* Corresponding author.
E-mail address: cho@bwh.harvard.edu

Cardiol Clin 37 (2019) 35–43
https://doi.org/10.1016/j.ccl.2018.08.003
0733-8651/19/© 2018 Elsevier Inc. All rights reserved.

further screening. Successful incorporation of genetic testing into clinical practice requires an understanding of the process and results to ensure appropriate interpretation by physicians and fully informed patients. Genetic testing is best accomplished in a specialized center with the necessary expertise, but all providers caring for patients with HCM should be literate in core genetic concepts.[5]

THE HYPERTROPHIC CARDIOMYOPATHY CLINIC TEAM

The care of families with HCM requires a multidisciplinary team that can address all aspects of the patient's clinical care, including genetics. Collaboration with genetics providers (genetic counselors or medical geneticists), ideally those familiar with cardiovascular genetics, is advised. Specialized HCM centers increasingly have a genetic counselor as part of the HCM clinic team or may collaborate with the genetics department within their institution. Moreover, to provide family-centered care, collaboration between adult and pediatric HCM providers is ideal to allow continuity of care across the lifespan and a consistent management approach within the family.

GENETIC COUNSELING

As defined by the National Society of Genetic Counselors, genetic counseling is "the process of helping people understand and adapt to the medical, psychological and familial implications of genetic contributions to disease." Although genetic counseling can be provided by a variety of health care providers with appropriate knowledge and expertise, genetic counselors have specialized training in the genetic basis and psychological impact of disease. They play a valuable role in the management of patients and families with genetic disease by helping patients understand and adjust to information that impacts not only themselves, but also their families.

Genetic counseling includes the acquisition and assessment of family history, patient education about the genetic basis of disease and genetic testing options, assistance with family communication, and psychological support. The educational needs of the patient may evolve over time and should be revisited periodically. For example, a person diagnosed with HCM as an adolescent would benefit from genetic counseling in adulthood to review reproductive implications at a time when the information is more relevant.

One component of genetic counseling is a detailed discussion about available genetic testing. Key elements of the genetic testing discussion, detailed in later discussion, form the basis of the informed consent process by providing patients with information about the benefits, uses, and limitations of genetic testing. Through this process, patients gain the information needed to understand how genetic testing may impact their care and the care of their families.

CLINICAL USES OF GENETIC TESTING

Genetic testing can be divided into 2 distinct categories: diagnostic testing and predictive testing. *Diagnostic testing* is used to identify the genetic cause of disease in a person with HCM. This information can confirm a suspected diagnosis and, importantly, differentiate HCM from phenocopies. Several disorders have cardiac features that overlap with HCM, such as Fabry disease and cardiac amyloidosis, but may have different inheritance patterns, additional systemic manifestations, or alternate treatment strategies that impact patient and family management. Furthermore, emerging evidence suggests that the presence of a sarcomere variant portends worse outcomes (increased risks for atrial fibrillation and heart failure) compared with HCM patients with unknown genetic or other causes.[6,7] In the future, more refined understanding of genotype-phenotype correlations may allow for targeted disease management and anticipatory guidance.

Identifying the genetic cause of disease in a patient also allows for targeted genetic testing of at-risk relatives to better define their risk of developing disease. This process of predictive testing is often referred to as cascade screening because it begins by testing the first-degree relatives of an affected individual and then broadens, or cascades, to include the first-degree relatives of anyone in the family who subsequently tests positive (**Fig. 1**).

Predictive testing consists of very focused testing looking for a specific DNA variant and is used to determine whether a relative inherited the DNA variant presumed to be the cause of disease in the family. Those who test positive, meaning they carry the pathogenic DNA variant, are at risk for disease development and should continue with recommended longitudinal surveillance. These individuals also have a 50% chance of transmitting the variant to each of their children. Relatives who test negative for the DNA variant can be reassured that they are not at risk for developing HCM or transmitting risk to their offspring. If there is a high level of confidence that the DNA variant is the definitive cause of disease in the family, they are typically dismissed from serial screening. However, they are advised to present for evaluation if there is any clinical change. Recent guidelines suggest baseline cardiac

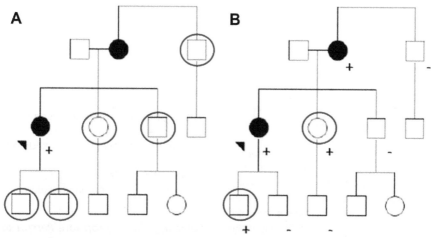

Fig. 1. Predictive genetic screening. Circles denote women; boxes denote men. Shaded symbols have a clinical diagnosis of HCM; clear symbols denote clinically unaffected status. The proband (marked with an *arrow*) has positive genetic test results with a pathogenic sarcomere variant identified (+). (*A*) The circled relatives each have a 50% chance of carrying the same pathogenic variant identified in the proband. These relatives are at risk for having unrecognized HCM or for developing HCM. Longitudinal clinical screening is recommended for these individuals to assess for clinical disease expression. (*B*) The results of cascade screening. The 2 individuals denoted by circled clear symbols and (+) carry the pathogenic sarcomere variant and are at risk for HCM. These individuals should undergo longitudinal clinical screening. By contrast, the individuals denoted by clear symbols and (−) do not carry the pathogenic variants. These individuals and their offspring are not at risk for HCM and do not require longitudinal clinical screening.

evaluation of at-risk relatives who are pursuing predictive genetic testing, even if genetic test results are negative.[2] This comprehensive approach to family evaluation will define the presence or absence of HCM in each family member at baseline, which enhances the ability to assess segregation and, importantly, to detect nonsegregation (family member with HCM who does not have the variant), which suggests that the variant may not be pathogenic or that there may be a second variant in the family (**Fig. 2**).

Certain patient and family characteristics increase the likelihood that genetic testing will yield valuable information:

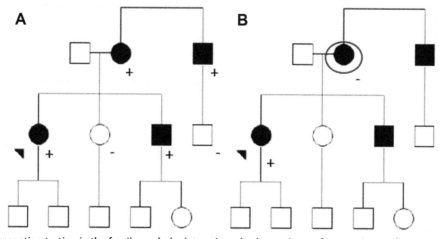

Fig. 2. Segregation testing in the family can help determine whether variants of uncertain significance (VUS) are disease causing. (*A*) The clinically affected proband (marked with an *arrow*) has a VUS (+). More information is required before the variant can be used for predictive testing in other relatives. Other affected family members (*shaded symbols*) can be tested to determine if they carry the variant. In this family, the variant segregates with disease and is present in 3 other affected relatives. In (*B*) the variant found in the clinically affected proband (marked with an *arrow*) does not segregate with disease because it is not present in an affected relative (*circle*). If the diagnosis of HCM is accurate in that relative, this finding indicates that the variant does not cause HCM in this family.

- *Familial disease*: Evidence of familial disease has been shown to increase the pretest probability of a positive result from approximately 30% to greater than 50%.[8,9]
- *Diagnostic certainty*: Patients with atypical patterns of hypertrophy (ie, apical) and/or other potential triggers for hypertrophy (ie, hypertension, intense athletic conditioning) are less likely to have positive genetic testing results.[10]
- *Available family members*: Having affected family members available for genetic testing enables segregation analysis to gain additional evidence and confidence that an identified variant is the cause of disease in a family. Furthermore, the presence of clinically unaffected family members who are interested in predictive testing increases the potential clinical utility of testing, because these results can directly impact medical management.

Taken together, it is possible to identify scenarios that depict varying levels of diagnostic yield and clinical utility (**Fig. 3**). For example, a patient with a characteristic pattern of asymmetric septal hypertrophy, a family history of HCM, and at-risk relatives interested in predictive testing represents a high-yield, high-clinical-utility scenario. By contrast, a person with an equivocal diagnosis, no affected relatives for segregation, and no first-degree relatives would represent a low-yield, low-clinical-utility scenario. Predictive scores and models have also been proposed to estimate the likelihood of positive results and could be considered

when deciding whether to pursue genetic testing.[11,12]

THE GENETIC TESTING PROCESS

There are many steps in the genetic testing process (**Fig. 4**):

1. Select the appropriate person to test
2. Choose the appropriate test
3. Perform pretest counseling and obtain informed consent
4. Review and disclose results
5. Facilitate family communication

Selecting the Appropriate Person to Test

Begin by generating a 3-generation family history, or pedigree, to illustrate family relationships and relevant medical history. Careful phenotyping and review of family members' medical records are often critical to confirm diagnoses, cause of death, and other patient-reported health information. A detailed pedigree helps to not only assess for familial disease but also identify the preferred genetic testing proband and allows visualization of at-risk relatives who might use predictive genetic testing to define their risk of disease development. The proband selected for genetic testing is ideally the most severely affected person in the family, identified by the extent of disease progression and/or age of onset and adverse outcomes experienced. Multiple sarcomere variants are found in ~3% to 5% of patients who may exhibit severe HCM: massive hypertrophy and/or early onset and recurrent adverse

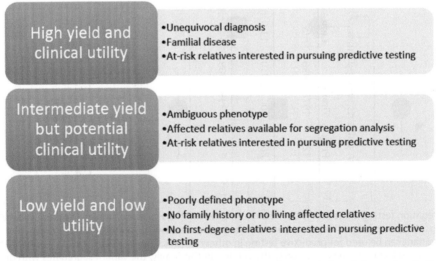

High yield and clinical utility	•Unequivocal diagnosis •Familial disease •At-risk relatives interested in pursuing predictive testing
Intermediate yield but potential clinical utility	•Ambiguous phenotype •Affected relatives available for segregation analysis •At-risk relatives interested in pursuing predictive testing
Low yield and low utility	•Poorly defined phenotype •No family history or no living affected relatives •No first-degree relatives interested in pursuing predictive testing

Fig. 3. Factors influencing the yield and utility of genetic testing. Characteristics of the patient's diagnosis and family history can help to differentiate situations whereby genetic testing might have greater benefit from those situations whereby genetic testing is less likely to yield helpful information.

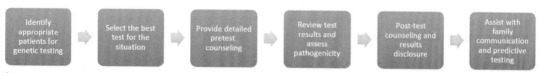

Fig. 4. Steps in the genetic testing process. Genetic testing is a multistep process, and depending on the outcome steps, such as variant interpretation and test selection, results, and testing strategy may need to be revisited over time.

outcomes. As such, selecting the most severely affected person can potentially identify multiple relevant variants that may be present individually or collectively in family members.[13,14] Although testing may begin with one individual, the proband, it is useful to confirm positive results in affected individuals in the family to establish certainty that the genetic cause is identified. Therefore, genetic testing should often be considered a family-based test.

Choosing the Appropriate Test

Although there are many different methodologies for genetic testing, HCM genetic testing is most often accomplished using multigene panels. The composition of the panels will vary by laboratory but consistently include sarcomere genes with strong evidence that they cause HCM. These genes include myosin binding protein C (*MYBPC3*), myosin heavy chain (*MYH7*), cardiac troponin T (*TNNT2*), cardiac troponin I (*TNNI3*), alpha-tropomyosin (*TPM1*), myosin essential and regulatory light chains (*MLY2*, *MYL3*), and cardiac actin (*ACTC*). Genes causing well-characterized phenocopies of HCM (ie, *GLA* for Fabry disease) are also typically included. Panels often include additional genes that have not been clearly proven to cause HCM. The clinical relevance of variants identified in these genes is thus often unclear. Available evidence suggests that increasing panel size does not necessarily lead to an increase in the likelihood of identifying a disease-causing mutation, although the likelihood of obtaining ambiguous results is increased.[8,14] Therefore, when there is a well-characterized phenotype, it is reasonable to order an HCM-specific multigene panel that focuses on genes with a stronger association to the phenotype and includes at least the 8 core sarcomere genes.

Broader genetic testing approaches, like whole exome sequencing and whole genome sequencing, are emerging, although like large multigene panels, these broad tests may not significantly improve clinically relevant detection rates. Furthermore, broader genetic testing introduces the possibility of incidental findings (genetic variants that are clinically actionable but unrelated to HCM) that may identify risk for other heritable conditions such as cancer.[15] Pretest counseling is particularly important when broad genetic

analyses are planned so as to discuss the potential for unanticipated findings that may cause psychological harm and the need for additional medical evaluations. However, broad genetic testing platforms do offer the promise that the vast data obtained from these tests may be beneficial over time because these datasets can be reanalyzed as new knowledge emerges.

Pretest Counseling and Informed Consent

Pretest and posttest counseling are essential parts of the genetic testing process. Pretest counseling informs the patient about important aspects of genetic testing, such as the potential implications of results for the patient and family, possible adverse psychosocial sequelae, the probabilistic rather than deterministic nature of genetic testing, and the potential for variant reclassification. Thorough pretest genetic counseling allows the patient to make an informed decision about whether to proceed with testing.

Results Review and Interpretation

The most challenging part of genetic testing is determining the pathogenicity of a variant–is this variant the cause of disease. This challenge is due in part to the complexity of the human genome and the lack of robust functional studies to demonstrate that a given variant has physiologic effect. A genetic testing laboratory's classification of a variant reflects their assessment of the probability that the variant is the cause of disease, based on available data. Guidelines put forth by the American College of Medical Genetics and Genomics (ACMG) and the Association for Molecular Pathology provide a framework for variant interpretation by outlining the categories of data that should be factored into this assessment and the relative strength of that data.[16] Examples of data sources include the frequency of the variant in affected individuals and the general population, functional and computational data, known disease mechanisms, and segregation of the variant in the family. As gene-specific knowledge evolves, these criteria may be further refined, as was recently shown with the *MYH7* gene.[17] In recent years, publicly available tools like Clinvar,[18] ClinGen,[19] Exac,[20] and Gnomad[20] (**Table 1**) have aided the overall variant

Table 1
Variant interpretation resources

Resource	Information Provided	Web Address
ClinVar	Variant classifications ± supporting data from contributing laboratories	www.clinvar.com
ClinGen	Curated data about the association between specific genes and variants and phenotype	www.clinicalgenome.org/
ExAC	Population-based variant frequency from exome sequencing	http://exac.broadinstitute.org/
gnomAD	Population-based variant frequency from exome and genome sequencing	http://gnomad.broadinstitute.org/
CardioClassifier	Interactive data interpretation tool	https://www.cardioclassifier.org/

interpretation process by promoting data sharing between laboratories and providing aggregated population frequency data from large-scale sequencing efforts. Most laboratories use a 5-tier classification system: benign, likely benign, uncertain significance, likely pathogenic, and pathogenic (**Table 2**).

Pathogenic and likely pathogenic variants are considered positive results. Pathogenic variants define the cause of the disease and can be used for predictive testing in family members who are at risk for disease development. Likely pathogenic variants have less certainty for causing disease, but may be clinically actionable. Discretion is

Table 2
Genetic test results and their clinical implications

	Genetic Test Result				
	Negative		**Uncertain**	**Positive**	
Variant classification	Benign or no variant found	Likely benign	VUS	Likely pathogenic	Pathogenic
Meaning	No important variants detected; genetic disease cannot be excluded	Variant detected is likely harmless; genetic disease cannot be excluded	Ambiguous result May be reclassified if additional information becomes available	Variant is likely responsible for causing HCM Family segregation studies may provide additional evidence for causality	Variant is responsible for causing HCM
Utility for proband	None	None	Unknown	Likely suggests HCM diagnosis May inform management or lead to additional diagnostic studies	Establishes HCM diagnosis May inform management
Utility for family	Predictive testing is unavailable, rely on phenotypic evaluations	Predictive testing is unavailable, rely on phenotypic evaluations	Predictive genetic testing is not advised, but testing affected relatives for segregation may be informative	Predictive genetic testing of unaffected relatives should be approached carefully and may be combined with phenotypic evaluation	Can be used for predictive genetic testing

Adapted from Cirino AL, Harris S, Lakdawala NK, et al. Role of genetic testing in inherited cardiovascular disease: a review. JAMA Cardiol 2017;2(10):1157; with permission.

needed when using likely pathogenic variants for predictive testing in family members.

Variants of uncertain significance (VUS) are ambiguous results that do not define the genetic cause of disease and cannot be used for predictive testing. Here, again, knowledge of family history can be a valuable tool. Studying other affected relatives enables segregation studies to help determine if the variant is a reliable marker of disease risk in the family (see **Fig. 2**). The more affected relatives, and particularly distantly related affected relatives, found to carry the variant, the more likely it is that the variant is the cause of disease. Conversely, the absence of the variant in just one relative with a definitive diagnosis of HCM is a strong indication that the variant alone is not the cause of HCM in the family. Segregation analysis can be a valuable step for any variant but particularly for VUS because these additional data may lead to a reclassification from VUS to pathogenic/likely pathogenic or likely benign.

Likely benign and benign results are considered negative and are typically not reported by the laboratory. A negative result does not exclude the possibility of genetic disease; it simply indicates that a genetic cause was not identified among the genes evaluated. Therefore, family screening may still be appropriate, particularly if there is evidence of famililal disease, and broader genetic testing could be considered at that time or in the future as available tests and knowledge evolve.

Because variant classification is based on evidence available at the time of analysis, the classification can change over time as new data emerge. This possibility lies in stark contrast to most laboratory testing where the value or result of a test is not expected to vary over time.[21,22] Laboratory policies for updating ordering providers about classification updates vary. Thus, clinicians must be aware of laboratory policies and develop a strategy for remaining abreast of updates and managing this information. Some reclassifications will necessitate recontacting the patient, potentially after significant time has elapsed, to revise recommendations previously made to families. For example, if a variant of uncertain significance is upgraded to likely pathogenic or pathogenic, predictive testing may now be an option for family members. Conversely, if a pathogenic variant is downgraded to uncertain significance, relatives who were previously released from ongoing surveillance may need to resume recommended screening.

Family Communication

Genetic testing is a family-based test because the impact of the results extends beyond the individual patient. Because of privacy restrictions, providers cannot directly contact at-risk relatives to share genetic test results that may be important for their health. Instead, communication must be funneled through the genetic testing proband. Many factors can impact the effectiveness of this communication, including family dynamics, gender, proband knowledge, and current health of the proband.[23] Providers play an important role in the communication process by first assuring their patient's understanding of the information and then providing guidance and resources for the proband to share information with at-risk family members.[24] A common example of such a resource is a family letter that is written by the provider and includes relevant information for family members. Despite these efforts, the uptake of recommended family screening is suboptimal, which suggests that other strategies may be necessary.[25,26] Furthermore, the dynamic nature of variant interpretation means that a provider's relationship with a patient, and family, could extend beyond the time that the patient is under that provider's care.

IMPORTANT CONSIDERATIONS WITH GENETIC TESTING

Genetic testing differs from traditional laboratory testing in several ways. As previously discussed, the results are probabilistic in nature and may be revised over time, requiring a provider to revisit some steps in the genetic testing process, such as results disclosure and facilitation of family communication. Careful consideration must be given to predictive testing in young children. Professional societies such as the ACMG and the National of Genetic Counselors have position statements recommending against predictive genetic testing of minors for adult onset disease. HCM is not exclusively adult onset, and therefore, it does not squarely fall under this guidance, but the age-dependent penetrance of HCM makes the timing of predictive testing a relevant consideration. The principle arguments against testing minors are that it removes their autonomy to make this decision for themselves when they reach the age of majority; there is the potential for negative psychological sequelae for those who test positive; and there are no currently available treatments that prevent or modify disease.[27]

In addition, for all unaffected at-risk relatives, there is the potential for genetic discrimination. In the United States, the Genetic Information Nondiscrimination Act of 2008 was enacted to provide protection against discrimination by health insurers and employers. With this law, genetic information and family history cannot be used to unfavorably bias decisions regarding employment or health insurance. However, the provisions of this legislation do not extend to providers of life insurance, disability, or long-term care insurance. Similar legal protections exist in other countries as well. A person undergoing predictive genetic testing should be informed of potential discrimination risks as part of the consent process to allow the individual to determine their personal level of concern. For some, securing the desired insurance before proceeding with clinical screening or genetic testing is the preferred strategy.

Genetic testing can also be used for reproductive planning by testing a current pregnancy or undergoing preimplantation genetic diagnosis (PGD). PGD is done in conjunction with in vitro fertilization to perform genetic testing on a single cell extracted from early-stage embryos. Only embryos without the familial variant are implanted to achieve pregnancy. Interest in reproductive genetic testing is highly personal, and those interested should be referred to specialty reproductive genetics clinics for a more detailed discussion to further facilitate decision-making.

TEST LOGISTICS

Genetic testing is more accessible than it was in years past. Logistical details of genetic testing can vary by laboratory, but overall, the process has become faster and less expensive. Those who may have declined genetic testing in the past solely for financial reasons could reconsider genetic testing now, because out-of-pocket costs for most patients have declined substantially. Peripheral blood is still the preferred source of DNA but, increasingly, alternate DNA sources, such as saliva, buccal swab, and dried blood spot cards, are acceptable, and sample collection may be done remotely.

SUMMARY

HCM genetic testing allows for a more refined, gene-based diagnosis that may guide patient management and assist with the definitive identification of at-risk relatives now. Furthermore, genetic testing offers the potential for more targeted treatment in the future. It is important to recognize that genetic testing requires additional considerations and counseling beyond traditional laboratory testing. Collaboration with, or referral to, specialized clinics is essential when incorporating genetic testing into clinical practice to achieve optimal outcomes for the patient and their family.

REFERENCES

1. Gersh BJ, Maron BJ, Bonow RO, et al. 2011 ACCF/AHA guideline for the diagnosis and treatment of hypertrophic cardiomyopathy: a report of the American College of Cardiology Foundation/American Heart Association Task Force on Practice Guidelines. Circulation 2011;124(24):e783–831.
2. Hershberger RE, Givertz MM, Ho CY, et al. Genetic evaluation of cardiomyopathy-a heart failure society of America practice guideline. J Card Fail 2018;24(5):281–302.
3. Elliott PM, Anastasakis A, Borger MA, et al. 2014 ESC guidelines on diagnosis and management of hypertrophic cardiomyopathy: the task force for the diagnosis and management of hypertrophic cardiomyopathy of the European Society of Cardiology (ESC). Eur Heart J 2014;35(39):2733–79.
4. van Velzen HG, Schinkel AFL, Baart SJ, et al. Outcomes of contemporary family screening in hypertrophic cardiomyopathy. Circ Genom Precis Med 2018;11(4):e001896.
5. Mital S, Musunuru K, Garg V, et al. Enhancing literacy in cardiovascular genetics: a scientific statement from the American Heart Association. Circ Cardiovasc Genet 2016;9(5):448–67.
6. Ingles J, Burns C, Bagnall RD, et al. Nonfamilial hypertrophic cardiomyopathy: prevalence, natural history, and clinical implications. Circ Cardiovasc Genet 2017;10(2) [pii:e001620].
7. Ho C, Day S, Ashley E, et al. Genotype and lifetime burden of disease in hypertrophic cardiomyopathy: insights from the Sarcomeric Human Cardiomyopathy Registry (SHaRe). Circulation 2018. [Epub ahead of print].
8. Alfares AA, Kelly MA, McDermott G, et al. Results of clinical genetic testing of 2,912 probands with hypertrophic cardiomyopathy: expanded panels offer limited additional sensitivity. Genet Med 2015;17(11):880–8.
9. Ingles J, Sarina T, Yeates L, et al. Clinical predictors of genetic testing outcomes in hypertrophic cardiomyopathy. Genet Med 2013;15(12):972–7.
10. Bos JM, Will ML, Gersh BJ, et al. Characterization of a phenotype-based genetic test prediction score for unrelated patients with hypertrophic cardiomyopathy. Mayo Clin Proc 2014;89(6):727–37.
11. Murphy SL, Anderson JH, Kapplinger JD, et al. Evaluation of the mayo clinic phenotype-based genotype predictor score in patients with clinically diagnosed hypertrophic cardiomyopathy. J Cardiovasc Transl Res 2016;9(2):153–61.
12. Gruner C, Ivanov J, Care M, et al. Toronto hypertrophic cardiomyopathy genotype score for prediction of a positive genotype in hypertrophic cardiomyopathy. Circ Cardiovasc Genet 2013;6(1):19–26.
13. Ingles J, Doolan A, Chiu C, et al. Compound and double mutations in patients with hypertrophic

cardiomyopathy: implications for genetic testing and counselling. J Med Genet 2005;42(10):e59.

14. Burns C, Bagnall RD, Lam L, et al. Multiple gene variants in hypertrophic cardiomyopathy in the era of next-generation sequencing. Circ Cardiovasc Genet 2017;10(4) [pii:e001666].

15. Cirino AL, Lakdawala NK, McDonough B, et al. A comparison of whole genome sequencing to multigene panel testing in hypertrophic cardiomyopathy patients. Circ Cardiovasc Genet 2017;10(5) [pii: e001768].

16. Richards S, Aziz N, Bale S, et al. Standards and guidelines for the interpretation of sequence variants: a joint consensus recommendation of the American College of medical genetics and Genomics and the association for Molecular Pathology. Genet Med 2015;17(5):405–24.

17. Kelly MA, Caleshu C, Morales A, et al. Adaptation and validation of the ACMG/AMP variant classification framework for MYH7-associated inherited cardiomyopathies: recommendations by ClinGen's inherited cardiomyopathy expert panel. Genet Med 2018;20(3):351–9.

18. Harrison SM, Riggs ER, Maglott DR, et al. Using ClinVar as a resource to support variant interpretation. Curr Protoc Hum Genet 2016;89:8, 16.1-8. 16.23.

19. Rehm HL, Berg JS, Brooks LD, et al. ClinGen–the clinical genome resource. N Engl J Med 2015; 372(23):2235–42.

20. Lek M, Karczewski KJ, Minikel EV, et al. Analysis of protein-coding genetic variation in 60,706 humans. Nature 2016;536(7616):285–91.

21. Das KJ, Ingles J, Bagnall RD, et al. Determining pathogenicity of genetic variants in hypertrophic cardiomyopathy: importance of periodic reassessment. Genet Med 2014;16(4):286–93.

22. Walsh R, Thomson K, Ware JS, et al. Reassessment of Mendelian gene pathogenicity using 7,855 cardiomyopathy cases and 60,706 reference samples. Genet Med 2017;19(2):192–203.

23. Batte B, Sheldon JP, Arscott P, et al. Family communication in a population at risk for hypertrophic cardiomyopathy. J Genet Couns 2015;24(2):336–48.

24. Forrest LE, Delatycki MB, Skene L, et al. Communicating genetic information in families–a review of guidelines and position papers. Eur J Hum Genet 2007;15(6):612–8.

25. Smagarinsky Y, Burns C, Spinks C, et al. Development of a communication aid for explaining hypertrophic cardiomyopathy genetic test results. Pilot Feasibility Stud 2017;3:53.

26. Miller EM, Wang Y, Ware SM. Uptake of cardiac screening and genetic testing among hypertrophic and dilated cardiomyopathy families. J Genet Couns 2013;22(2):258–67.

27. Charron P, Arad M, Arbustini E, et al. Genetic counselling and testing in cardiomyopathies: a position statement of the European society of Cardiology Working Group on Myocardial and Pericardial diseases. Eur Heart J 2010;31(22):2715–26.

Lifestyle Modification and Medical Management of Hypertrophic Cardiomyopathy

Stephen B. Heitner, MD*, Katherine L. Fischer, MSN, RN

KEYWORDS

- Cardiomyopathy • Hypertrophic • Beta-blocker • Calcium channel blocker • Disopyramide
- Ranolizine • Obstruction • Lifestyle

KEY POINTS

- Symptoms of obstructive hypertrophic cardiomyopathy are made more profound in the setting of comorbidities.
- Poor nutrition, a sedentary lifestyle, obesity, sleep-disordered breathing, anxiety, and depression are all significant, treatable, and frequently unaddressed issues facing patients with hypertrophic cardiomyopathy.
- Beta-blockers, calcium channel blockers, and the addition of disopyramide are all effective therapies for obstructive hypertrophic cardiomyopathy.
- Ranolazine can be considered as an additional therapy for treatment of angina or symptomatic premature ventricular contractions in hypertrophic cardiomyopathy.

INTRODUCTION

Hypertrophic cardiomyopathy (HCM), the most common monogenic cardiomyopathy, is a remarkably heterogeneous disease.[1] Despite the relatively high incidence and fascinating scientific history of this condition (see Julio A. Panza and Srihari S. Naidu's article, "Historical Perspectives in the Evolution of Hypertrophic Cardiomyopathy," in this issue), there remains only 1 drug labeled for its medical treatment in the United States, coupled with a scarcity of data on the impact of lifestyle choices on HCM (and vice versa).

Although there are no data supporting treating asymptomatic patients, it is important to consider that HCM is a slowly progressive condition and for patients whose symptoms remain inadequately treated, both quality of life and longevity will be adversely impacted. Conversely, patients treated aggressively and according to contemporary standards often enjoy a normal life expectancy and excellent overall quality of life.[2–8] As such, a very careful history, physical examination, and evaluation of imaging and exercise data are crucial.

Although therapies exist for many of the clinical manifestations of HCM, these have been dealt with in depth by authors of their respective sections (see Jason T. Jacobson's article, "Arrhythmia Evaluation and Management," and Avi Levine and colleagues' article, "Advanced Heart Failure Management and Transplantation," and Sei Iwai's article, "Sudden Cardiac Death Risk Stratification and the Role of the ICD," and Timothy C. Wong and Matthew Martinez's article, "Novel Pharmacotherapy for Hypertrophic

Disclosure Statement: S.B. Heitner has received a moderate degree of funding for research and consulting from MyoKardia. K.L. Fischer has no disclosures to report.
Department of Cardiology, OHSU Hypertrophic Cardiomyopathy Center, Knight Cardiovascular Institute, Oregon Health & Science University, 3181 Southwest Sam Jackson Park Road, UHN62, Portland, OR 97239, USA
* Corresponding author.
E-mail address: Heitner@ohsu.edu

Cardiol Clin 37 (2019) 45–54
https://doi.org/10.1016/j.ccl.2018.08.004

Cardiomyopathy," in this issue). This article details the medical therapies currently available for the treatment of obstructive HCM (oHCM) and our understanding of potential impact for lifestyle modification in patients with oHCM and nonobstructive HCM.

LIFESTYLE MODIFICATION

Therapeutic interventions in HCM tend to target the symptoms and prevention of complications. Although medications and procedures (such as septal myectomy and alcohol septal ablation) are the mainstay treatments for oHCM, there is increasing evidence of the importance of lifestyle modification that may result in a similar effect, and perhaps even alter the disease course.

Diet and Nutrition

Considering the well-documented and temporal relationship between the quantity and composition of nutrition on the degree of obstruction[9] and the impact of dehydration (preload),[10] it comes as no surprise that many individuals with oHCM frequently report subjective changes in symptomatology in accordance with dietary changes. Patients may note exacerbation of symptoms with carbohydrate-rich foods, large or rich meals, and alcohol ingestion.[11] Consequently, advising patients to eat smaller meals, restrict simple carbohydrates, avoid dehydration, limit alcohol consumption, and restrict postprandial physical activity may have tremendous impact on overall symptom burden. Although research validating these recommendations is limited, 1 study has shown that patients with obstruction who limit meal size and increase hydration tend to experience a decrease in symptoms and require less medication.[12]

Physical Activity

Recommendations regarding the degree, type, and frequency of exercise are one of the most controversial in the field, with disagreement in current expert consensus statements in the United States and Europe.[13–15] Current exercise guidelines focus on restrictions with the risk for sudden cardiac death (SCD) as a core consideration. This finding stems from early observations that many SCD victims succumbed during physical exertion[16] and that HCM was the leading cause of SCD in young athletes in the United States.[17] However, subsequent studies have challenged these findings and suggested that the estimated risk of SCD in athletes with HCM who compete in sports is in the range of 0.03% to 0.10% per year.[18] We now know that the majority of people with HCM who suffer an SCD event do so either at a time remote from exercise or while completely at rest.[19–21]

Although there is increasing evidence tipping the so-called exercise paradox[22] in favor of the cardioprotective benefits of exercise, the safety net of the guidelines in the absence of data perpetuates recommendations to restrict activity. The tragic, and often public, nature of sudden death in athletes promotes anxiety in both patients and providers, further promoting a very conservative approach to exercise and a focus in research on SCD prevention. Consequently, patients with HCM frequently report purposefully reducing or even ceasing meaningful exercise after their diagnosis, and that exercise restriction has a significant negative impact on their emotional well-being.[23] This finding is particularly true for patients diagnosed at a young age or who are asymptomatic.[24]

Patients with HCM engage in recreational and moderate intensity activity less often and for shorter periods than the general population,[10,23] and most do not meet the minimum health promotion guidelines for physical activity with nearly 90% of patients being considered insufficiently active.[25] Patients with HCM also feel out of shape, have a higher incidence of obesity, and report exercise restrictions negatively impact quality of life.[23] Factors being seen as a barrier to exercise in patients with HCM also include a higher body mass index, beta-blocker use, higher New York Heart Association functional class, other medical comorbidities, and lower socioeconomic status.[25]

When looking at this from the perspective of population health, patients with HCM are unlikely to achieve the minimum activity recommendations for cardiovascular health,[25] which begs the question of whether patients with HCM may benefit more from guidelines that focus on activity recommendations rather than restrictions.[26] To date, no research has demonstrated detrimental effects of recreational or moderate intensity exercise in patients with HCM and there is no evidence that higher intensity athletic training accelerates the HCM phenotype.[10,25,27] In fact, moderate intensity personalized exercise programs have been shown to improve objective measures of health, including heart rate recovery, functional capacity measured by metabolic equivalents, exercise duration, exercise capacity as measured by peak V_{O_2}, and subjective clinical condition and physical functioning.[28,29] Importantly, moderate intensity exercise was shown to be safe and with no evidence of disease progression, increased arrhythmias, or other adverse outcomes,[27–29] supporting a paradigm shift aimed at providing patients with HCM with evidence-based recommendations for rather than against regular exercise. Lifestyle and Exercise in HCM (LIVE-HCM), a prospective observational study, will hopefully provide insight for developing exercise recommendations that can aid in patient–provider shared decision making.

Obesity

The coexistence of obesity and HCM represents a complex interplay, and often a downward spiral of symptoms, psychological well-being, and treatment options. Whether obesity is a result of poor nutritional choices, physical limitations owing to heart failure or obstruction, or caused by lack of physical exercise, the importance of attempting to maintain a healthy body mass cannot be overstated. Moreover, the presence of obesity is independently associated with more frequent and severe symptoms (dyspnea, chest pain). Obese patients with a similar HCM phenotype have higher resting and provoked gradients when compared with nonobese patients.[30,31] Obese patients also have lower exertional capacity and are more likely to progress to severe heart failure.[31] This pattern results in patients with comorbid obesity and symptomatic HCM being more frequently resistant to medical therapy. Consideration for advanced therapies (septal reduction therapies and heart transplantation) is complicated by the presence of significant obesity, physical incapacity, and the cascade of comorbidities that are part and parcel of this syndrome (obstructive sleep apnea, diabetes mellitus, higher postoperative infection rates, etc). Because of the complexity of the presentation of obesity in HCM, it is best practice to address obesity (or the potential for obesity) early. This strategy requires the expertise of a skilled, multidisciplinary team consisting of a dietician, an expert in lifestyle modification in the obese, a cardiovascular behavioral therapist, and referral for bariatric surgery if indicated.

Sleep-Disordered Breathing

Poor sleep quality is reported in 32% to 80% of patients with HCM, significantly more frequently than in the non-HCM population.[32–34] HCM has also been shown to be an independent predictor of poor sleep quality after controlling for other factors.[35] Comorbid sleep-disordered breathing (SDB) and HCM has a similar profile to comorbid obesity and HCM. Although SDB is correlated with obesity in patients with and without HCM, patients with HCM and SDB tend to be less obese than patients with SDB and no HCM,[33] suggesting that obesity is not the only driver of SDB in HCM.

The impact of SDB in patients with HCM is seemingly profound. There are higher estimated cardiac filling pressures[36–38] and possible associated adverse cardiac remodeling.[34] Patients with HCM with SDB have more severe symptoms, a worse self-reported quality of life,[32,34,35] and severe functional impairment; 56% of patients with HCM with SDB achieve less than 60% of predicted Vo_2 peak compared with 34% of patients with HCM without SDB.[37,38] As in the general population, patients with SDB and HCM have a greater degree of hypertension[32] and a higher prevalence of atrial fibrillation.[32,33,36,38] Although the treatment of SDB improves hypertension and there is anecdotal evidence that it may improve heart failure symptoms,[32] more research is needed to confirm these outcomes and to investigate whether treatment reduces the prevalence of atrial fibrillation and what role testing for SDB should play in the evaluation of patients with HCM.

Psychological Well-Being

Psychological well-being as a component of overall health-related quality of life has not been well-researched in patients with HCM. The available evidence suggests that depression and anxiety are common in patients with HCM,[39,40] and patients with HCM are more depressed than the general population,[39,41] but not as depressed as patients with coronary artery disease.[41] Surprisingly, there seems to be no correlation between SCD risk (collective risk or presence of individual risk factors) and depression, or between time since diagnosis and depression.[41] Emotional stress has been shown to trigger symptoms in about one-half of patients with HCM, making emotional stress a less common trigger than exertion, but a more common trigger than eating a meal or lying flat, with chest pain being the most commonly reported emotionally triggered symptom.[42] Although the HCM population as a whole reports fairly high physical, emotional and overall quality of life, patients with symptoms or comorbidities report lower quality of life.[41,43] Patients who report emotionally triggered symptoms have a lower quality of life than patients who experience exercise-triggered symptoms.[42] The relationship between mental well-being and symptoms may represent another example of a self-perpetuating cycle in which symptoms impact mental well-being and mental well-being impacts symptoms.[42]

Providers should be acutely aware that there is a deep and immeasurable psychological impact as a direct result of the hereditary nature of HCM. The decision to undergo genetic testing is often associated with concern for family members, and can be abetted by support of extended family or laden with pressure for or against testing.[24] Although the majority of patients who undergo testing report complete satisfaction with the decision to test, those who test positive report greater uncertainty and distress, and less positive impact from the results than those who test negative.[44]

In families that undergo cascade genetic testing, there will undoubtedly be family members identified as gene positive and phenotype negative (silent gene carriers). The psychological impact on silent gene carriers is not well-researched, but an extreme range in response has been observed, from those who are completely unconcerned to those with significant anxiety.[24] Family planning and life insurance are issues of particular concern for some gene carriers, whether the HCM phenotype is expressed or not.[24,44] The lack of research indicating how silent gene carriers should be treated, including regarding activity restrictions, adds to the potential psychological impact. Conversely, individuals who are gene negative for HCM are relieved from serial testing and potential anxiety over phenotype progression.

Patients with HCM are frequently young, considering or already having children of their own, and are anxious about their future. Moreover, some patients come from a background where they have lost 1 or more relatives to SCD, heart failure, stroke, or who have undergone cardiac transplantation. Patients, particularly the young, are considering the potential for life-long medications, implantable defibrillators, appropriate and inappropriate implantable cardioverter-defibrillator discharges, and the possibility of open heart surgery. The best practice is multidisciplinary and offers consultation with both a cardiovascular behavioral therapist and cardiovascular genetic counselor for all patients, both of which have been gratefully accepted by many individuals (**Fig. 1**).

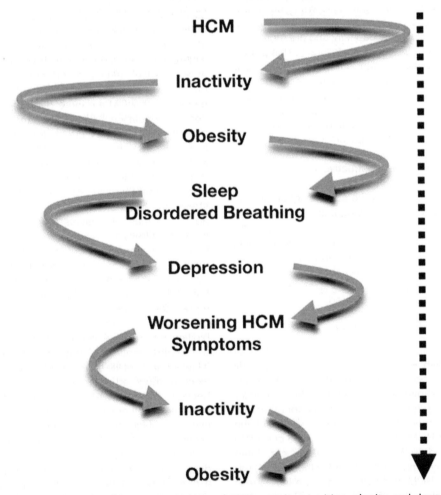

Fig. 1. The downward spiral and interconnectedness of HCM, exercise, nutrition, obesity, and sleep-disordered breathing. HCM, hypertrophic cardiomyopathy.

PHARMACOTHERAPIES

Symptoms are the primary driver for initiation of pharmacotherapy in patients. The exception is the pediatric age group where symptoms may not be reliable, and it is acceptable to use physical examination and echocardiographic findings to establish the need to start a drug. Patients with nonobstructive HCM and heart failure with preserved left ventricular function should be managed with diuretics for symptom control. Those who develop systolic dysfunction (heart failure with reduced ejection fraction) should be treated according to current evidence-based medical therapy for heart failure; this topic is discussed in Avi Levine and colleagues' article, "Advanced Heart Failure Management and Transplantation," in this issue. Additionally, it should be noted that several clinical trials in the recent past have sought to evaluate the efficacy in symptom alleviation and improvement of exertional capacity (losartan,[45] spironolactone,[46] ranolazine,[47] eleclazine,[48] and perhexiline), but have failed. Currently, there are ongoing studies

evaluating valsartan[49] and mavacamten[50,51] in the various phenotypes and stages of HCM. A global algorithm for standard treatment options is included in **Figs. 2** and **3**.

Beta-Blockers

Nonvasodilating beta-blockers (propranolol, metoprolol, atenolol) were the first class of drug shown to be effective in oHCM and, to date, propranolol is the only drug currently labeled for use in oHCM.[52] Beta-blockers are usually the first-line drugs to treat symptomatic oHCM and have been shown, albeit with limited strength of evidence, to alleviate some symptoms and potentially improve exercise tolerance in individuals able to tolerate them.[53,54] Patients should be counseled about the potential for central nervous system side effects (fatigue, depression and erectile dysfunction) but advised to trial the therapy for several weeks as patients can acclimate to these side effects. Further, bradycardia, hypotension, and exacerbation of reactive airways disease should be considered.

Drug	Class	Effect on LVOTO	Effect on Angina	Dose Range	Common Side Effects
Metoprolol tartrate or Metoprolol succinate	Cardio-selective β-blocker	↓↓	↓↓↓	25–200 mg bid or 400 mg daily	Fatigue, depression, erectile dysfunction, bradycardia, hypotension, asthma exacerbation
Propranolol or Propranolol ER	Non-selective β-blocker	↓↓	↓↓↓	20–40 mg tid/qid or 80–160 mg daily	
Verapamil or Verapamil ER	Non-dihydropyridine CCB	↓↓	↓↓	40–160 mg tid or 120–480 mg daily	Constipation, bradycardia, hypotension
Diltiazem or Diltiazem ER	Non-dihydropyridine CCB	↓↓	↓↓	30–90 mg qid or 120–480 mg daily	
Disopyramide or Disopyramide ER	Class 1A antiarrhythmic	↓↓↓	↓↓↓	100–200 mg tid/qid or 100–300 mg bid	Dry eyes, dry mouth, constipation, urinary retention, blurred vision, QTc prolongation
Ranolazine	Late-sodium channel blocker	-	↓↓↓	500–1000 mg bid	Dizziness, confusion, constipation, blurred vision, QTc prolongation

Fig. 2. The most commonly used medical therapies for symptomatic hypertrophic cardiomyopathy (HCM). Included is the drug class, effect on left ventricular outflow tract obstruction (LVOTO), angion, their commonly used dose range, and most frequently encountered side effects. CCB, calcium channel blocker; ER, extended release.

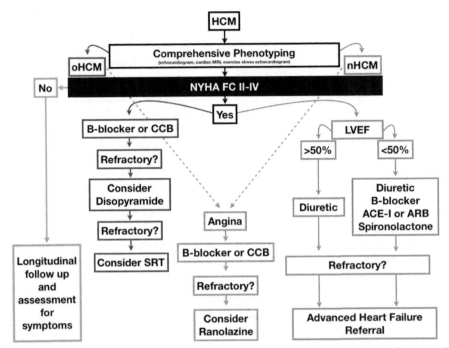

Fig. 3. Basic algorithm for the institution of conventional medical therapy in symptomatic hypertrophic cardio-myopathy (HCM). For a detailed review of either arrhythmia management or advance heart failure management, please refer to Jason T. Jacobson's article, "Arrhythmia Evaluation and Management," and Avi Levine and colleagues' article, "Advanced Heart Failure Management and Transplantation," respectively, in this issue. ACE-I, angiotensin converting enzyme inhibitor; ARB, angiotensin receptor blocker; CCB, calcium channel blocker; LVEF, left ventricular ejection fraction; nHCM, nonobstructive hypertrophic cardiomyopathy; oHCM, obstructive hypertrophic cardiomyopathy; SRT, septal reduction therapy. (*Data from* Gersh BJ, Maron BJ, Bonow RO, et al. 2011 ACCF/AHA guideline for the diagnosis and treatment of hypertrophic cardiomyopathy: executive summary: a report of the American College of Cardiology Foundation/American Heart Association Task Force on Practice Guidelines. J Am Col Cardiol 2011;58(25):2703–38; and Elliott PM, Anastasakis A, Borger AM, et al. 2014 ESC guidelines on diagnosis and management of hypertrophic cardiomyopathy: the task force for the diagnosis and management of hypertrophic cardiomyopathy of the European Society of Cardiology (ESC). Euro Heart J 2014;35(39):2733–79.)

In general, long-acting formulations given in twice daily format are used in the treatment of outflow tract obstruction, with propranolol and metoprolol being the best-studied beta-blockers. Although long-acting formulations are preferred, metoprolol tartrate used twice daily is a low cost beta-blocker that is usually well-tolerated. Beta-blockers with alpha-blocking activity (carvedilol, labetalol, bisoprolol, nebivolol) can theoretically aggravate the left ventricular outflow tract obstruction and in general should be avoided in oHCM with the exception being patients with comorbid systemic hypertension; we have had success in careful institution of one of these agents with concomitant control of both oHCM symptoms and hypertension.

Calcium Channel Blockers

It is common practice to trial beta-blockers initially, and if ineffective or not well-tolerated, to initiate a nondihydropyradine calcium channel blocker (verapamil or diltiazem). Recently, there is a suggestion based on analysis of claims data that patients treated with calcium channel blockers had fewer adverse outcomes than those treated with beta-blockers.[55] Moreover, diltiazem may have a potential disease-modifying effect in a subset of patients.[56] Thus, it may be preferable to begin medical therapy with diltiazem as the first agent, although this strategy is not yet supported by the guidelines documents.

Dihydropyridine calcium channel blockers (eg, nifedipine, amlodipine, nicardipine, felodipine), and to a much lesser extent nondihydropyridine calcium channel blockers at high doses[57] may exacerbate obstruction owing to their afterload-reducing properties and as a result should be avoided. Similar to beta-blockers, calcium channel blockers primarily ameliorate provokable, as opposed to resting, gradients. Calcium channel blockers should not be used in patients with congestive heart failure or significant pulmonary hypertension because these drugs may exacerbate the condition. Again, potential side effects should be discussed with patients (constipation particularly with verapamil; bradycardia and hypotension) before initiating therapy.

Disopyramide

Disopyramide is a class I antiarrhythmic drug with negative inotropic properties, making it a useful drug to treat patients with symptomatic oHCM.[58–61] As opposed to beta-blockers and calcium channel blockers, disopyramide can decrease both resting and provokable obstruction. Disopyramide can successfully ameliorate symptoms of exertional shortness of breath, angina, presyncope, and syncope in up to two-thirds of patients with oHCM.[62]

Disopyramide is generally well-tolerated, although its anticholinergic side effects can limit its tolerability. For the commonest side effects of dry mouth and dry eyes, patients should be advised to drink more fluids and use artificial tears if needed. Blurred vision and urinary retention, which can occur in both men and women, are more troublesome and may result in discontinuation of therapy. One can consider the addition of pyridostigmine for side effect control, although we do not have specific experience with this. Importantly, disopyramide should always be given together with an atrioventricular nodal blocker (beta-blocker or calcium channel blocker) because the anticholinergic effects can theoretically enhance conduction through the atrioventricular node, resulting in very high ventricular response rates, and even ventricular fibrillation, in the setting of atrial fibrillation. Disopyramide has the potential to be proarrhythmic and has QT-prolonging properties, so many providers recommend starting therapy as an inpatient, with dose titration and evaluation of the QTc regularly. Our practice is to introduce disopyramide as an outpatient and have routine monitoring of the electrocardiogram for QTc prolongation. The onset of the drug effect is short; the majority of responders report alleviation of symptoms within 24 to 48 hours. One observational study suggests that this agent is safe, effective, and may also be associated with a survival advantage.[58]

Ranolazine

Ranolazine is an antianginal agent that is approved by the US Food and Drug Administration that acts through inhibition of the late sodium current and through its effect on adenosine release. In HCM, as well as in myocardial ischemia and congestive heart failure, there is an association with enzyme-induced sodium-channel phosphorylation[63] that disrupts sodium channel inactivation and increases the late sodium current activity.

Although there was a suggestion from basic research that late sodium current inhibition would improve exercise capacity and relieve symptoms in nonobstructive HCM, this finding was not confirmed in clinical trials.[63] Ranolazine has been shown to be safe and effective at treating angina in the HCM population, and as such is a very useful adjunct for angina that is refractory to either beta-blockers or calcium channel blockers.[64] Further, the use of ranolazine (in HCM and non-HCM cohorts) is associated with less ventricular ectopy.[65] Although this has not been translated into improved clinical outcomes, ranolazine may also be useful in patients with symptomatic premature ventricular contractions.

SUMMARY

Nutrition, a sedentary lifestyle, obesity, SDB, anxiety, and depression are all significant, modifiable, and frequently unaddressed issues facing patients with HCM. Additionally, the symptoms of oHCM are made more profound in the setting of these comorbidities and lifestyle issues. Beta-blockers, calcium channel blockers, and disopyramide are all effective therapies for oHCM, and ranolazine can be considered as an additional therapy for the treatment of angina or symptomatic premature ventricular contractions in HCM. Patients with refractory symptoms should be considered for the appropriate septal reduction procedure if feasible.

REFERENCES

1. Maron BJ, Rowin EJ, Maron MS. Global burden of hypertrophic cardiomyopathy. JACC Heart Fail 2018;6(5):376–8.
2. Maron MS, Olivotto I, Betocchi S, et al. Effect of left ventricular outflow tract obstruction on clinical outcome in hypertrophic cardiomyopathy. N Engl J Med 2003;348(4):295–303.
3. Maron BJ, Rowin EJ, Udelson JE, et al. Clinical spectrum and management of heart failure in hypertrophic cardiomyopathy. JACC Heart Fail 2018;6(5):353–63.
4. Maron BJ, Casey SA, Poliac LC, et al. Clinical course of hypertrophic cardiomyopathy in a regional United States cohort. JAMA 1999;281(7):650–5.
5. Cecchi F, Olivotto I, Montereggi A, et al. Hypertrophic cardiomyopathy in Tuscany: clinical course and outcome in an unselected regional population. J Am Coll Cardiol 1995;26(6):1529–36.

6. Spirito P, Chiarella F, Carratino L, et al. Clinical course and prognosis of hypertrophic cardiomyopathy in an outpatient population. N Engl J Med 1989; 320(12):749–55.

7. Cannan CR, Reeder GS, Bailey KR, et al. Natural history of hypertrophic cardiomyopathy. A population-based study, 1976 through 1990. Circulation 1995;92(9):2488–95.

8. Maron BJ, Casey SA, Haas TS, et al. Hypertrophic cardiomyopathy with longevity to 90 years or older. Am J Cardiol 2012;109(9):1341–7.

9. Feiner E, Arabadjian M, Winson G, et al. Post-prandial upright exercise echocardiography in hypertrophic cardiomyopathy. J Am Coll Cardiol 2013; 61(24):2487–8.

10. Finocchiaro G, Magavern E, Sinagra G, et al. Impact of demographic features, lifestyle, and comorbidities on the clinical expression of hypertrophic cardiomyopathy. J Am Heart Assoc 2017;6(12) [pii: e007161].

11. Paz R, Jortner R, Tunick PA, et al. The effect of the ingestion of ethanol on obstruction of the left ventricular outflow tract in hypertrophic cardiomyopathy. N Engl J Med 1996;335(13):938–41.

12. Kansal MM, Mookadam F, Tajik AJ. Drink more, and eat less: advice in obstructive hypertrophic cardiomyopathy. Am J Cardiol 2010;106(9):1313–6.

13. Maron BJ, Chaitman BR, Ackerman MJ, et al. Recommendations for physical activity and recreational sports participation for young patients with genetic cardiovascular diseases. Circulation 2004;109(22): 2807–16.

14. Gersh BJ, Maron BJ, Bonow RO, et al. 2011 ACCF/AHA guideline for the diagnosis and treatment of hypertrophic cardiomyopathy: executive summary: a report of the American College of Cardiology Foundation/American Heart Association task force on practice guidelines. J Am Coll Cardiol 2011;58(25): 2703–38.

15. Authors/Task Force Members, Elliott PM, Anastasakis A, et al. 2014 ESC guidelines on diagnosis and management of hypertrophic cardiomyopathy: the task force for the diagnosis and management of hypertrophic cardiomyopathy of the European Society of Cardiology (ESC). Eur Heart J 2014;35(39):2733–79.

16. Teare D. Asymmetrical hypertrophy of the heart in young adults. Br Heart J 1958;20(1):1–8.

17. Maron BJ, Shirani J, Poliac LC, et al. Sudden death in young competitive athletes. Clinical, demographic, and pathological profiles. JAMA 1996; 276(3):199–204.

18. Alpert C, Day SM, Saberi S. Sports and exercise in athletes with hypertrophic cardiomyopathy. Clin Sports Med 2015;34(3):489–505.

19. Maron BJ, Doerer JJ, Haas TS, et al. Sudden deaths in young competitive athletes: analysis of 1866 deaths in the United States, 1980-2006. Circulation 2009;119(8):1085–92.

20. Maki S, Ikeda H, Muro A, et al. Predictors of sudden cardiac death in hypertrophic cardiomyopathy. Am J Cardiol 1998;82(6):774–8.

21. Corrado D, Basso C, Rizzoli G, et al. Does sports activity enhance the risk of sudden death in adolescents and young adults? J Am Coll Cardiol 2003; 42(11):1959–63.

22. Maron BJ. The paradox of exercise. N Engl J Med 2000;343(19):1409–11.

23. Reineck E, Rolston B, Bragg-Gresham JL, et al. Physical activity and other health behaviors in adults with hypertrophic cardiomyopathy. Am J Cardiol 2013;111(7):1034–9.

24. Bonner C, Spinks C, Semsarian C, et al. Psychological impact of a positive gene result for asymptomatic relatives at risk of hypertrophic cardiomyopathy. J Genet Couns 2018;27(5):1040–8.

25. Sweeting J, Ingles J, Timperio A, et al. Physical activity in hypertrophic cardiomyopathy: prevalence of inactivity and perceived barriers. Open Heart 2016; 3(2):e000484.

26. Saberi S, Day SM. Exercise and hypertrophic cardiomyopathy: time for a change of heart. Circulation 2018;137(5):419–21.

27. Dejgaard LA, Haland TF, Lie OH, et al. Vigorous exercise in patients with hypertrophic cardiomyopathy. Int J Cardiol 2018;250:157–63.

28. Saberi S, Wheeler M, Bragg-Gresham J, et al. Effect of moderate-intensity exercise training on peak oxygen consumption in patients with hypertrophic cardiomyopathy: a randomized clinical trial. JAMA 2017;317(13):1349–57.

29. Klempfner R, Kamerman T, Schwammenthal E, et al. Efficacy of exercise training in symptomatic patients with hypertrophic cardiomyopathy: results of a structured exercise training program in a cardiac rehabilitation center. Eur J Prev Cardiol 2015;22(1): 13–9.

30. Canepa M, Sorensen LL, Pozios I, et al. Comparison of clinical presentation, left ventricular morphology, hemodynamics, and exercise tolerance in obese versus nonobese patients with hypertrophic cardiomyopathy. Am J Cardiol 2013; 112(8):1182–9.

31. Olivotto I, Maron BJ, Tomberli B, et al. Obesity and its association to phenotype and clinical course in hypertrophic cardiomyopathy. J Am Coll Cardiol 2013;62(5):449–57.

32. Konecny T, Somers VK. Sleep-disordered breathing in hypertrophic cardiomyopathy: challenges and opportunities. Chest 2014;146(1):228–34.

33. Nerbass FB, Pedrosa RP, Danzi-Soares NJ, et al. Obstructive sleep apnea and hypertrophic cardiomyopathy: a common and potential harmful combination. Sleep Med Rev 2013;17(3):201–6.

34. Prinz C, Bitter T, Oldenburg O, et al. Incidence of sleep-disordered breathing in patients with hypertrophic cardiomyopathy. Congest Heart Fail 2011; 17(1):19–24.

35. Pedrosa RP, Lima SG, Drager LF, et al. Sleep quality and quality of life in patients with hypertrophic cardiomyopathy. Cardiology 2010;117(3):200–6.

36. Konecny T, Brady PA, Orban M, et al. Interactions between sleep disordered breathing and atrial fibrillation in patients with hypertrophic cardiomyopathy. Am J Cardiol 2010;105(11):1597–602.

37. Konecny T, Geske JB, Ludka O, et al. Decreased exercise capacity and sleep-disordered breathing in patients with hypertrophic cardiomyopathy. Chest 2015;147(6):1574–81.

38. Aggarwal S, Jan MF, Agarwal A, et al. Hypertrophic cardiomyopathy associated with sleep apnea: serious implications and cogent management strategy. Expert Rev Cardiovasc Ther 2015;13(3): 277–84.

39. Morgan JF, O'Donoghue AC, McKenna WJ, et al. Psychiatric disorders in hypertrophic cardiomyopathy. Gen Hosp Psychiatry 2008;30(1):49–54.

40. Ingles J, Lind JM, Phongsavan P, et al. Psychosocial impact of specialized cardiac genetic clinics for hypertrophic cardiomyopathy. Genet Med 2008;10(2): 117–20.

41. Igoumenou A, Alevizopoulos G, Anastasakis A, et al. Depression in patients with hypertrophic cardiomyopathy: is there any relation with the risk factors for sudden death? Heart Asia 2012;4(1):44–8.

42. Lampert R, Salberg L, Burg M. Emotional stress triggers symptoms in hypertrophic cardiomyopathy: a survey of the Hypertrophic Cardiomyopathy Association. Pacing Clin Electrophysiol 2010;33(9): 1047–53.

43. Christiaans I, van Langen IM, Birnie E, et al. Quality of life and psychological distress in hypertrophic cardiomyopathy mutation carriers: a cross-sectional cohort study. Am J Med Genet A 2009; 149a(4):602–12.

44. Wynn J, Holland DT, Duong J, et al. Examining the psychosocial impact of genetic testing for cardiomyopathies. J Genet Couns 2018;27(4):927–34.

45. Axelsson A, Iversen K, Vejlstrup N, et al. Efficacy and safety of the angiotensin II receptor blocker losartan for hypertrophic cardiomyopathy: the INHERIT randomised, double-blind, placebo-controlled trial. Lancet Diabetes Endocrinol 2015; 3(2):123–31.

46. Maron MS, Chan RH, Kapur NK, et al. Effect of spironolactone on myocardial fibrosis and other clinical variables in patients with hypertrophic cardiomyopathy. Am J Med 2018;131(7):837–41.

47. Olivotto I, Camici PG, Merlini PA, et al. Efficacy of ranolazine in patients with symptomatic hypertrophic cardiomyopathy: the RESTYLE-HCM randomized,

double-blind, placebo-controlled study. Circ Heart Fail 2018;11(1):e004124.

48. Elliott PM. Evolving story of clinical trials in hypertrophic cardiomyopathy. Circ Heart Fail 2018;11(1): e004572.

49. Ho CY, McMurray JJV, Cirino AL, et al. The design of the valsartan for attenuating disease evolution in early sarcomeric hypertrophic cardiomyopathy (VANISH) trial. Am Heart J 2017;187: 145–55.

50. Clinical study to evaluate mavacamten (MYK-461) in adults with symptomatic obstructive hypertrophic cardiomyopathy (EXPLORER-HCM). (ClinicalTrials.gov Identifier: NCT03470545). Available at: https://clinicaltrial.gov. Accessed July 16, 2018.

51. A phase 2 study of mavacamten in adults with symptomatic non-obstructive hypertrophic cardiomyopathy (nHCM) (MAVERICK-HCM) (ClinicalTrials.gov Identifier: NCT03442764). Available at: https://clinicaltrial.gov. Accessed July 16, 2018.

52. Cherian G, Brockington IF, Shah PM, et al. Beta-adrenergic blockade in hypertrophic obstructive cardiomyopathy. Br Med J 1966;1(5492):895–8.

53. Adelman AG, Shah PM, Gramiak R, et al. Long-term propranolol therapy in muscular subaortic stenosis. Br Heart J 1970;32(6):804–11.

54. Flamm MD, Harrison DC, Hancock EW. Muscular subaortic stenosis. Prevention of outflow obstruction with propranolol. Circulation 1968;38(5): 846–58.

55. Gombar S, Moneghetti KJ, Callahan A, et al. Beta-blockers inferior to calcium channel blockers in hypertrophic cardiomyopathy [abstract: 21307]. Circulation 2017;136(Suppl 1):A21307.

56. Ho CY, Lakdawala NK, Cirino AL, et al. Diltiazem treatment for pre-clinical hypertrophic cardiomyopathy sarcomere mutation carriers: a pilot randomized trial to modify disease expression. JACC Heart Fail 2015;3(2):180–8.

57. Epstein SE, Rosing DR. Verapamil: its potential for causing serious complications in patients with hypertrophic cardiomyopathy. Circulation 1981;64(3): 437–41.

58. Sherrid MV, Barac I, McKenna WJ, et al. Multicenter study of the efficacy and safety of disopyramide in obstructive hypertrophic cardiomyopathy. J Am Coll Cardiol 2005;45(8):1251–8.

59. Pollick C, Kimball B, Henderson M, et al. Disopyramide in hypertrophic cardiomyopathy. I. Hemodynamic assessment after intravenous administration. Am J Cardiol 1988;62(17):1248–51.

60. Pollick C. Disopyramide in hypertrophic cardiomyopathy. II. Noninvasive assessment after oral administration. Am J Cardiol 1988;62(17):1252–5.

61. Pollick C. Muscular subaortic stenosis: hemodynamic and clinical improvement after disopyramide. N Engl J Med 1982;307(16):997–9.

62. Louie EK, Edwards LC 3rd. Hypertrophic cardiomyopathy. Prog Cardiovasc Dis 1994;36(4): 275–308.

63. Coppini R, Ferrantini C, Yao L, et al. Late sodium current inhibition reverses electromechanical dysfunction in human hypertrophic cardiomyopathy. Circulation 2013;127(5):575–84.

64. Gentry JL 3rd, Mentz RJ, Hurdle M, et al. Ranolazine for treatment of angina or dyspnea in hypertrophic cardiomyopathy patients (RHYME). J Am Coll Cardiol 2016;68(16):1815–7.

65. Bazoukis G, Tse G, Letsas KP, et al. Impact of ranolazine on ventricular arrhythmias - A systematic review. J Arrhythm 2018;34(2):124–8.

Arrhythmia Evaluation and Management

Jason T. Jacobson, MD, FHRS

KEYWORDS

- Hypertrophic cardiomyopathy • Pacemakers • Ventricular arrhythmias • Atrial fibrillation • Stroke

KEY POINTS

- Patients with atrial fibrillation and hypertrophic cardiomyopathy require anticoagulation.
- An apical position is best for right ventricular pacing in patients with hypertrophic cardiomyopathy.
- Monomorphic ventricular tachycardia is mostly seen in hypertrophic cardiomyopathy in the dilated phase or when an apical aneurysm is present.
- Patients with sustained ventricular arrhythmias and hypertrophic cardiomyopathy require an implantable cardioverter-defibrillator.

ARRHYTHMIA EVALUATION

The identification of arrhythmia in patients with hypertrophic cardiomyopathy (HCM) is of great importance. Although the standard 12-lead electrocardiogram aids in the diagnosis of HCM and active arrhythmia, it does little for arrhythmia screening. Holter monitors can identify frequent arrhythmia or happen to fortuitously capture infrequent arrhythmias in the 24 to 72 hours that they are used. They also can provide statistical data regarding heart rates for assessment of medical therapy (β-blockers, calcium channel blockers) effects on sinus and atrioventricular (AV) nodal function, or ventricular rates during atrial fibrillation (AF). They are not a good option for capturing paroxysmal arrhythmias over the long term. Event monitors and mobile cardiac outpatient telemetry can be used for up to 4 weeks and are better suited to detect episodes of nonsustained ventricular tachycardia for risk stratification or paroxysmal AF, as well as investigate symptoms of palpitations, presyncope or syncope. The advent of the implantable loop recorder has revolutionized outpatient monitoring, allowing for up to 3 years of constant monitoring with a device that is injected just under the skin. These devices also allow for remote monitoring via a base station or smartphone application, allowing for the clinician to be alerted for detected arrhythmias at least daily. The 2011 American College of Cardiology Foundation (ACCF)/American Heart Association (AHA) HCM guidelines recommend an initial 24-hour Holter monitor to investigate for ventricular tachyarrhythmias (VTA) (Class I), AF (Class IIb), and evaluate symptoms of palpitations or light headedness (Class I), and repeat Holter monitoring every 1 to 2 years to evaluate for VTA (Class IIa).[1] These guidelines do not comment on long-term monitoring; however, the European Society of Cardiology recommends to perform 48-hour Holter monitoring (Class I) as an initial assessment and routinely every 12 to 24 months (or 6–12 months if the left atrial diameter is ≥45 mm), and to investigate palpitations and syncope, and to consider an implantable loop recorder for the evaluation of syncope (Class IIa) and palpitations (Class IIb) if electrocardiographic monitoring has been unrevealing.[2]

The use of invasive electrophysiology studies in HCM is limited to those undergoing ablation for supraventricular tachyarrhythmias (SVTA) or VTA and has no place in general for risk stratification of sudden cardiac death (SCD).[1,2]

Disclosures: Consultant-Abbott Medical, Atricure; Speaker-Biotronik; Research Funding-Abbott Medical.
Complex Arrhythmia Ablation Program, New York Medical College, Westchester Medical Center, Macy 130, 100 Woods Road, Valahalla, NY 10595, USA
E-mail address: Jason.Jacobson@wmchealth.org

Cardiol Clin 37 (2019) 55–62
https://doi.org/10.1016/j.ccl.2018.08.005
0733-8651/19/

BRADYCARDIA AND PACING

Although patients with HCM may develop sinus and AV nodal dysfunction (de novo and medical therapy induced), a review of permanent pacemaker (PPM) indications is beyond the scope of this article. However, the unique physiology of HCM does require special consideration in regards to ventricular pacing. Additionally, septal reduction therapies, both alcohol septal ablation (ASA) and surgical myectomy (SM), pose specific risks to the conduction system.

Septal Reduction and Conduction

The risk to the bundle branches depends on the technique undertaken. Myectomy is generally undertaken from the basal left ventricular (LV) septum, in close proximity to the proximal left bundle branch. Whereas left bundle branch block (LBBB) is the concern with SM, ASA jeopardizes the right bundle branch (RBB), because the proximal septal perforating arteries supply this structure most frequently. In multiple series of SM, about 47% developed new LBBB, whereas only 2% developed right BBB (RBBB).[3,4] Similarly, RBBB was seen in 37% to 40% of patients undergoing ASA (**Fig. 1**), but no LBBB developed acutely.[4,5]

Complete AV block (CAB) can occur transiently with both procedures; however, PPM implantation is not necessary in all cases. With modern ASA techniques, about 20% of patients will experience intraprocedural CAB.[6] Many will recover acutely, and the rate of delayed (>48 hours) CAB and PPM implantation has been reported to be 9% to 25%,[6–9] with the highest reported rates coming from the earliest studies. As expected from the data regarding development of BBB during ASA/SM, those with preexisting LBBB undergoing ASA and those with preexisting RBBB undergoing SM have a high risk of CAB.[4,7] In the previously mentioned SM cohorts, only 3% required PPM for CAB.[3,4] A recent metaanalysis found a PPM rate of 10% with ASA and 4% with SM.[10]

Left Ventricular Outflow Tract Obstruction

Patients with symptomatic LV outflow tract obstruction (LVOTO) refractory to medical therapy may find relief by the dyssynchronous contraction pattern induced by ventricular pacing. Early work focused on atrial triggered right ventricular apical (RVA) pacing, which facilitated a decrease in LVOTO via asynchronous, paradoxic septal motion, in effect pulling the basal septum out of the way during contraction.[11–14] This process effectuates changes that lead to negative inotropy,[15] LV

dilation, and wall thinning,[16] as well as decreased septal anterior motion of the mitral valve.[11–14]

Early observational reports suggested a significant benefit of RVA pacing for LVOTO.[11–14,17] However, the M-Pathy trial, the first randomized trial of pacing for LVOTO, called this therapeutic option into question. The trial randomized 48 patients in an initially blinded, 3-month crossover study. All patients received dual chamber PPM and split into 2 treatment arms: initial dual chamber (DDD) pacing for 3 months followed by atrial pacing for another 3 months, and initial atrial pacing followed by DDD after 3 months. After the first 6 months of blinded crossover pacing, all patients were programmed to DDD pacing, unblinded. During the blinded phase, no difference was seen between groups in measures of symptoms or exercise capacity, including New York Heart Association functional class, quality of life score, treadmill exercise time, or peak oxygen consumption. After the 6 months of unblinded DDD pacing, the investigators found a 40% decrease in LVOT gradient and improvements in functional class and quality of life; however, no difference in peak oxygen consumption was seen.[18] A subset of patients older than 65 years did show improved functional capacity. Much of the symptomatic improvement after the unblinded pacing phase was ascribed to placebo effect.[18] Despite the small study size and a short duration of blinded treatment, which was followed by unblinded treatment, M-Pathy cast a dark shadow over RVA pacing as a treatment modality for LVOTO. This finding led to RVA pacing to being given a Class IIa indication in patients that have a DDD device for non-HCM indications (ACCF/AHA)[1] and a Class IIb indication for those who are medically refractory and suboptimal candidates for septal reduction therapy (ACCF/AHA and European Society of Cardiology).[1,2]

Although the enthusiasm for ventricular pacing was dampened, it was not completely wiped out. Subsequent studies have suggested that it takes more than 3 months to realize the benefits of RVA pacing, as can be seen after ASA.[19,20] Lucon and colleagues[19] followed patients for a median of 11.5 years and noted a progressive decrease in functional class, LVOT gradient (79 mm Hg baseline to 8 mm Hg at last follow-up), and presence of systolic anterior motion of the mitral valve (96% baseline, 15% at last follow-up). Jurado Román and colleagues[20] found similar results after median 8.5 years follow-up, albeit less impressive (eg, gradient 94.5 mm Hg to 35.9 mm Hg). Additionally, recent studies have investigated the effects of biventricular pacing on LVOTO. It is important to understand that this does not

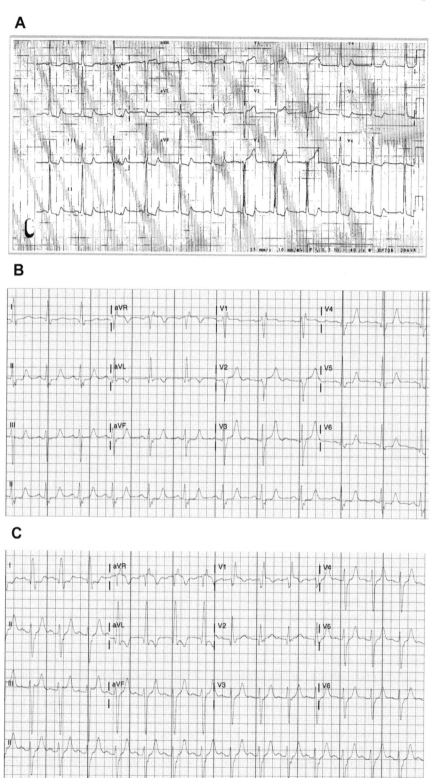

Fig. 1. Development of right bundle branch block (RBBB) after alcohol septal ablation (ASA). (*A*) Baseline electrocardiogram tracing shows a narrow QRS complex. (*B*) After ASA, RBBB is noted with anterior ST-segment elevations and a normal QRS axis. (*C*) After 4 days, q waves are seen in the anterior leads and the QRS axis has shifted, consistent with left anterior fascicular block. Later that day, complete heart block developed and a permanent pacemaker was implanted.

constitute cardiac "resynchronization therapy" in that biventricular pacing still induces dyssynchrony in the setting of normal His-Purkinje system function. An approach of biventricular pacing implantation with optimization of LVOT gradient reduction based on paced chamber (right ventricular, LV, and biventricular pacing) and AV node ablation (if necessary to allow for fully paced rhythm) has shown promise in early studies, out to 1 year.[21,22] Future studies will need to be randomized, blinded, and of sufficient duration to determine if biventricular pacing is truly effective. Of interest, in contradistinction, cardiac resynchronization therapy in patients with HCM who develop standard indications has not shown clear benefit in a small, observational study.[23]

SUPRAVENTRICULAR TACHYARRHYTHMIAS

Patients with HCM can experience the same SVTA as the general population. The management for the paroxysmal SVT (AV nodal reentry, AV reentry, and focal atrial tachycardia) is much the same. It is important to note that 2 glycogen storage disorders can mimic HCM and present with Wolf-Parkinson-White syndrome. These are genetic conditions owing to mutations in either the PRKAG2 or LAMP2 genes.[24,25] A full discussion of these disorders is not within the scope of this article. However, the sequelae and management of AF and atrial flutter are particular in HCM.

The incidence of clinically apparent AF in HCM is up to 22% in some series and increases with the duration of follow-up; 5% at diagnosis,[26] 10% by 5 years,[26] and 22% at 9 years,[27] with a yearly incidence of 2% per year.[27] In these, two-thirds were paroxysmal. When considering patients with HCM with PPM and an implantable cardioverter-defibrillator, an additional 24% (7%/year) asymptomatic patients can be identified.[28] When compared with the general population, the incidence of AF is 5-fold higher with HCM, with an attendant 2 to 4 times increase in mortality.[29,30]

With greater dependence on LV preload, patients with HCM may not tolerate the loss of atrial kick during AF/atrial flutter and the poor LV filling owing to rapid ventricular rates. In general, the treatment approach is similar to that for the general population and rests on the 3 pillars of rate control, stroke prophylaxis, and rhythm control.

Rate control is generally achieved with the same agents as are used first-line for LVOTO, β-blockers and nondihyrdopyridine calcium channel blockers.[1,2] Digitalis is to be avoided owing to the positive inotropic effects and potential to worsen LVOTO.[2] Even with good rate control, patients with HCM may still feel the aforementioned

impact of AF/atrial flutter on preload and a rhythm control strategy would be preferred. When medical rate control fails, and a particular patient is not a candidate for or fails rhythm control (discussed elsewhere in this article), AV node ablation and PPM can be a viable treatment option.[2]

Stroke prophylaxis is quite important with HCM and is not approached in the same fashion as the general population. The usual stroke risk scoring systems, such as CHADS2 and CHA2DS2-Vasc, do not apply. Olivotto and colleagues[27] found a 14% incidence of nonfatal stroke and a 7% stroke-related death over 9 years. In a metaanalysis of 10 other studies, Guttmann and colleagues[31] identified a stroke incidence of 3.75% per year in the HCM AF population. Therefore, it is recommended that any HCM patient with AF/atrial flutter be anticoagulated.[1,2] Although there have been no randomized studies investigating the target-specific oral anticoagulants (dabigitran, rivaroxaban, apixaban, edoxaban), these agents have been incorporated into HCM management alongside warfarin.[1,2]

Rhythm control options include antiarrhythmic drugs, catheter ablation, and surgical ablation. The younger age of the HCM population makes the long-term side effects of amiodarone undesirable for many. However, this drugs is the most efficacious of antiarrhythmics with the lowest proarrhythmic risk, and therefore is often used, especially the short term. Owing to the significant LV hypertrophy, the class Ic antiarrhythmic drugs (flecainide and propafenone) are generally avoided, owing to the risk of proarrhythmia.[1,2] Disopyramide (class Ic) is an agent that has found a niche use in HCM, because it is a strong negative inotrope and can be helpful for symptomatic LVOTO as well as AF/atrial flutter; however, data are scarce.[1,2] The anticholinergic and QT-prolonging effects have limited its use. Sotalol is often considered[1,2] owing to its low toxicities (QT prolongation/proarrhythmia) and reasonable efficacy, as well as the symptomatic benefit of the β-blocker effects. Dofetilide has a similar class III effect, but without the β-blocker, and can be considered as well.[1] The other class III agent, dronedarone, has been suggested in the ACCF/AHA guidelines,[1] but its use has been discouraged by the European Society of Cardiology.[2]

Surgical AF ablation should be considered at the time of SM in patients with HCM with AF, but is rarely considered as a standalone option. Although there are many surgical techniques for AF management, that discussion is beyond the scope of this article. A recent single-center case series by Bogachev-Prokophiev and associates[32] found a 1-year AF-free success of 89% and

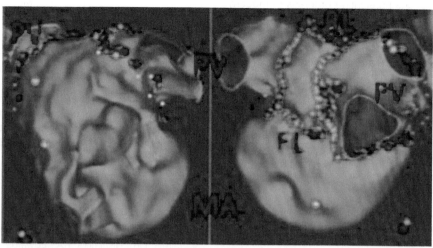

Fig. 2. Catheter ablation lesion set displayed on a 3-dimensional mapping system. Anteroposterior (*left*) and posteroanterior (*right*) views of radiofrequency ablation lesions (*pink and red spheres*) around the pulmonary veins (PV), as well as roof (RL) and floor (FL) lines to complete a box lesion isolating the posterior left atrial wall. MA, mitral annulus.

82.2% at 2 years in 45 patients. However, although patients were seen every 6 months, 72-hour Holter monitors were only obtained at 12 and 24 months. Additionally, the effect of SM alone on AF recurrence is not clear, making the reported success rate difficult to ascribe wholly to ablation.

Catheter ablation has gained widespread adoption for AF/atrial flutter in patients with varied heart disease. Typical cavotricuspid isthmus flutter is successfully treated with catheter ablation regardless of underlying heart disease with a long-term success rate exceeding 90%.[33] Catheter ablation for AF continues to evolve and success rates have improved with new techniques and technologies (**Fig. 2**). Although long-term success in patients with HCM is similar to that for the general population (paroxysmal, 71.8%; persistent, 47.5%),[34] this effect is achieved with a greater need for repeat procedures.[35–37] In a metaanalysis, Providencia and colleagues[37] found a 2-fold higher recurrence rate in patients with HCM compared with the general AF ablation population, with a greater need for antiarrhythmic drugs to help maintain sinus rhythm. Again, newer techniques and technologies are likely to change this equation.

VENTRICULAR ARRHYTHMIAS

The most dramatic presentation of HCM is SCD owing to VTA, most frequently ventricular fibrillation.[38] However, monomorphic ventricular tachycardia, both sustained and nonsustained ventricular tachycardia can be seen in patients with HCM.[38–40] In this issue, Sei Iwai's article,

"Sudden Cardiac Death Risk Stratification and the Role of the ICD," is devoted to this topic and, therefore, is not addressed here.

Ventricular fibrillation has classically been ascribed to myofibril disarray, which is a hallmark of HCM,[41] and is associated with altered gap junction distribution.[42] However, more recent pathologic[43] and MRI data suggest that scar deposition creates the substrate for VTA. This process is manifest as an increased risk of VTA and SCD with increasing burden of scar as evidenced by delayed enhancement on MRI.[44–46] This finding is not without correlate in other pathologies, including ischemic and nonischemic cardiomyopathies. Surviving perifibrosis myocardium may display differences in conduction velocity and refractory periods, leading to reentry, both functional (ventricular fibrillation, perhaps owing to the gap junction alterations in HCM[42]), and scar based (monomorphic ventricular tachycardia). Sustained monomorphic ventricular tachycardia is mostly seen in patients with either late-phase/dilated HCM and those with apical aneurysms/midcavity obstruction (**Fig. 3**). Sustained VTA can be triggered by moderate or more vigorous activity, SVTA, and premature ventricular contractions/nonsustained ventricular tachycardia.

Although an implantable cardioverter-defibrillator is the cornerstone of therapy in patients with HCM who experience sustained VTA, this device does not prevent recurrence, only SCD from the arrhythmia. Although there are no studies in patients with HCM, the mainstay of medical VTA therapy is with β-blockers. These

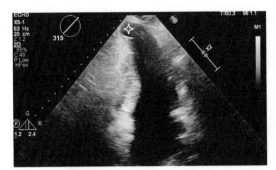

Fig. 3. Apical aneurysm (*star*) in a patient with monomorphic ventricular tachycardia.

agents not only may help to prevent adrenergic initiation of VTA, but also those initiated by rapid SVTA and premature ventricular contractions. For recurrent sustained VTA despite β-blocker, antiarrhythmic drugs are used next. The options are much the same as for AF; however, disopyramide is not used for VTA. Given the greater morbidity and potential mortality associated with VTA, the greater general efficacy of amiodarone for VTA makes it more difficult to forego.

For those patients with recurrent monomorphic ventricular tachycardia, catheter ablation is a viable option. The techniques used mimic those used for VT in the setting of prior myocardial infarction (identify scar via voltage mapping, identify circuit elements within the scar)[47,48]; however, patients with HCM often require epicardial mapping and ablation via a percutaneous subxyphoid approach.[49,50] This can yield a 78% freedom from implantable cardioverter-defibrillator shocks at 3 years.[51] Occasionally, patients with ventricular fibrillation have a premature ventricular contractions trigger of consistent morphology that can be mapped and ablated as well. Although there are no specific studies for this approach in HCM, case series of mixed populations have shown good results.[52]

SUMMARY

Arrhythmias, both supraventricular and ventricular, are a prominent feature of HCM. The timely detection and management is of the utmost importance to manage serious sequelae, such as stroke and sudden death. Although most therapies for arrhythmias in HCM parallel those in the general population, their applications have unique features in HCM that the treating clinician must appreciate.

REFERENCES

1. Gersh BJ, Maron BJ, Bonow RO, et al. 2011 ACCF/ AHA guideline for the diagnosis and treatment of hypertrophic cardiomyopathy: executive summary: a report of the American College of Cardiology Foundation/American Heart Association Task Force on practice guidelines. J Am Coll Cardiol 2011; 58(25):2703–38.

2. Authors/Task Force Members, Elliott PM, Anastasakis A, Borger MA, et al. 2014 ESC guidelines on diagnosis and management of hypertrophic cardiomyopathy: the task force for the diagnosis and management of hypertrophic cardiomyopathy of the European Society of Cardiology (ESC). Eur Heart J 2014;35(39):2733–79.

3. Wang S, Luo M, Sun H, et al. A retrospective clinical study of transaortic extended septal myectomy for obstructive hypertrophic cardiomyopathy in China. Eur J Cardiothorac Surg 2013;43(3):534–40.

4. Talreja DR, Nishimura RA, Edwards WD, et al. Alcohol septal ablation versus surgical septal myectomy: comparison of effects on atrioventricular conduction tissue. J Am Coll Cardiol 2004;44(12): 2329–32.

5. Liebregts M, Steggerda RC, Vriesendorp PA, et al. Long-term outcome of alcohol septal ablation for obstructive hypertrophic cardiomyopathy in the young and the elderly. JACC Cardiovasc Interv 2016;9(5):463–9.

6. Lawrenz T, Lieder F, Bartelsmeier M, et al. Predictors of complete heart block after transcoronary ablation of septal hypertrophy: results of a prospective electrophysiological investigation in 172 patients with hypertrophic obstructive cardiomyopathy. J Am Coll Cardiol 2007;49(24):2356–63.

7. Chang SM, Nagueh SF, Spencer WH 3rd, et al. Complete heart block: determinants and clinical impact in patients with hypertrophic obstructive cardiomyopathy undergoing nonsurgical septal reduction therapy. J Am Coll Cardiol 2003;42(2): 296–300.

8. El-Jack SS, Nasif M, Blake JW, et al. Predictors of complete heart block after alcohol septal ablation for hypertrophic cardiomyopathy and the timing of pacemaker implantation. J Interv Cardiol 2007; 20(1):73–6.

9. Schuller JL, Zipse MM, Krantz MJ, et al. Incidence and predictors of late complete heart block after alcohol septal ablation treatment of hypertrophic obstructive cardiomyopathy. J Interv Cardiol 2015; 28(1):90–7.

10. Liebregts M, Vriesendorp PA, Mahmoodi BK, et al. A systematic review and meta-analysis of long-term outcomes after septal reduction therapy in patients with hypertrophic cardiomyopathy. JACC Heart Fail 2015;3(11):896–905.

11. Fananapazir L, Epstein ND, Curiel RV, et al. Long-term results of dual-chamber (DDD) pacing in obstructive hypertrophic cardiomyopathy. Evidence for progressive symptomatic and hemodynamic

improvement and reduction of left ventricular hypertrophy. Circulation 1994;90(6):2731–42.

12. Jeanrenaud X, Goy JJ, Kappenberger L. Effects of dual-chamber pacing in hypertrophic obstructive cardiomyopathy. Lancet 1992;339(8805):1318–23.

13. Nishimura RA, Trusty JM, Hayes DL, et al. Dual-chamber pacing for hypertrophic cardiomyopathy: a randomized, double-blind, crossover trial. J Am Coll Cardiol 1997;29(2):435–41.

14. Slade AK, Sadoul N, Shapiro L, et al. DDD pacing in hypertrophic cardiomyopathy: a multicentre clinical experience. Heart 1996;75(1):44–9.

15. Pak PH, Maughan WL, Baughman KL, et al. Mechanism of acute mechanical benefit from VDD pacing in hypertrophied heart: similarity of responses in hypertrophic cardiomyopathy and hypertensive heart disease. Circulation 1998;98(3):242–8.

16. Yue-Cheng H, Zuo-Cheng L, Xi-Ming L, et al. Long-term follow-up impact of dual-chamber pacing on patients with hypertrophic obstructive cardiomyopathy. Pacing Clin Electrophysiol 2013;36(1):86–93.

17. Kappenberger L, Linde C, Daubert C, et al. Pacing in hypertrophic obstructive cardiomyopathy. A randomized crossover study. PIC Study Group. Eur Heart J 1997;18(8):1249–56.

18. Maron BJ, Nishimura RA, McKenna WJ, et al. Assessment of permanent dual-chamber pacing as a treatment for drug-refractory symptomatic patients with obstructive hypertrophic cardiomyopathy. A randomized, double-blind, crossover study (M-PATHY). Circulation 1999;99(22):2927–33.

19. Lucon A, Palud L, Pavin D, et al. Very late effects of dual chamber pacing therapy for obstructive hypertrophic cardiomyopathy. Arch Cardiovasc Dis 2013;106(6–7):373–81.

20. Jurado Román A, Montero Cabezas JM, Rubio Alonso B, et al. Sequential atrioventricular pacing in patients with hypertrophic cardiomyopathy: an 18-year experience. Rev Esp Cardiol (Engl Ed) 2016;69(4):377–83.

21. Berruezo A, Penela D, Burgos F, et al. Optimized pacing mode for hypertrophic cardiomyopathy: impact of ECG fusion during pacing. Heart Rhythm 2015;12(5):909–16.

22. Berruezo A, Vatasescu R, Mont L, et al. Biventricular pacing in hypertrophic obstructive cardiomyopathy: a pilot study. Heart Rhythm 2011;8(2):221–7.

23. Killu AM, Park JY, Sara JD, et al. Cardiac resynchronization therapy in patients with end-stage hypertrophic cardiomyopathy. Europace 2018;20(1):82–8.

24. Murphy RT, Mogensen J, McGarry K, et al. Adenosine monophosphate-activated protein kinase disease mimics hypertrophic cardiomyopathy and Wolff-Parkinson-White syndrome: natural history. J Am Coll Cardiol 2005;45(6):922–30.

25. Arad M, Maron BJ, Gorham JM, et al. Glycogen storage diseases presenting as hypertrophic cardiomyopathy. N Engl J Med 2005;352(4):362–72.

26. Robinson K, Frenneaux MP, Stockins B, et al. Atrial fibrillation in hypertrophic cardiomyopathy: a longitudinal study. J Am Coll Cardiol 1990;15(6):1279–85.

27. Olivotto I, Cecchi F, Casey SA, et al. Impact of atrial fibrillation on the clinical course of hypertrophic cardiomyopathy. Circulation 2001;104(21):2517–24.

28. Rowin EJ, Orfanos A, Estes NAM, et al. Occurrence and natural history of clinically silent episodes of atrial fibrillation in hypertrophic cardiomyopathy. Am J Cardiol 2017;119(11):1862–5.

29. Masri A, Kanj M, Thamilarasan M, et al. Outcomes in hypertrophic cardiomyopathy patients with and without atrial fibrillation: a survival meta-analysis. Cardiovasc Diagn Ther 2017;7(1):36–44.

30. van Velzen HG, Theuns DA, Yap SC, et al. Incidence of device-detected atrial fibrillation and long-term outcomes in patients with hypertrophic cardiomyopathy. Am J Cardiol 2017;119(1):100–5.

31. Guttmann OP, Rahman MS, O'Mahony C, et al. Atrial fibrillation and thromboembolism in patients with hypertrophic cardiomyopathy: systematic review. Heart 2014;100(6):465–72.

32. Bogachev-Prokophiev AV, Afanasyev AV, Zheleznev SI, et al. Concomitant ablation for atrial fibrillation during septal myectomy in patients with hypertrophic obstructive cardiomyopathy. J Thorac Cardiovasc Surg 2018;155(4):1536–42.e2.

33. Perez FJ, Schubert CM, Parvez B, et al. Long-term outcomes after catheter ablation of cavo-tricuspid isthmus dependent atrial flutter: a meta-analysis. Circ Arrhythm Electrophysiol 2009;2(4):393–401.

34. Zhao DS, Shen Y, Zhang Q, et al. Outcomes of catheter ablation of atrial fibrillation in patients with hypertrophic cardiomyopathy: a systematic review and meta-analysis. Europace 2016;18(4):508–20.

35. Bunch TJ, Munger TM, Friedman PA, et al. Substrate and procedural predictors of outcomes after catheter ablation for atrial fibrillation in patients with hypertrophic cardiomyopathy. J Cardiovasc Electrophysiol 2008;19(10):1009–14.

36. Di Donna P, Olivotto I, Delcre SD, et al. Efficacy of catheter ablation for atrial fibrillation in hypertrophic cardiomyopathy: impact of age, atrial remodelling, and disease progression. Europace 2010;12(3):347–55.

37. Providencia R, Elliott P, Patel K, et al. Catheter ablation for atrial fibrillation in hypertrophic cardiomyopathy: a systematic review and meta-analysis. Heart 2016;102(19):1533–43.

38. Maron BJ, Shen WK, Link MS, et al. Efficacy of implantable cardioverter-defibrillators for the prevention of sudden death in patients with hypertrophic cardiomyopathy. N Engl J Med 2000;342(6):365–73.

39. Furushima H, Chinushi M, Iijima K, et al. Ventricular tachyarrhythmia associated with hypertrophic cardiomyopathy: incidence, prognosis, and relation to type of hypertrophy. J Cardiovasc Electrophysiol 2010;21(9):991–9.

40. Ueda A, Fukamizu S, Soejima K, et al. Clinical and electrophysiological characteristics in patients with sustained monomorphic reentrant ventricular tachycardia associated with dilated-phase hypertrophic cardiomyopathy. Europace 2012;14(5):734–40.

41. Maron BJ, Roberts WC. Quantitative analysis of cardiac muscle cell disorganization in the ventricular septum of patients with hypertrophic cardiomyopathy. Circulation 1979;59(4):689–706.

42. Sepp R, Severs NJ, Gourdie RG. Altered patterns of cardiac intercellular junction distribution in hypertrophic cardiomyopathy. Heart 1996;76(5):412–7.

43. Varnava AM, Elliott PM, Mahon N, et al. Relation between myocyte disarray and outcome in hypertrophic cardiomyopathy. Am J Cardiol 2001;88(3):275–9.

44. Chan RH, Maron BJ, Olivotto I, et al. Prognostic value of quantitative contrast-enhanced cardiovascular magnetic resonance for the evaluation of sudden death risk in patients with hypertrophic cardiomyopathy. Circulation 2014;130(6):484–95.

45. Adabag AS, Maron BJ, Appelbaum E, et al. Occurrence and frequency of arrhythmias in hypertrophic cardiomyopathy in relation to delayed enhancement on cardiovascular magnetic resonance. J Am Coll Cardiol 2008;51(14):1369–74.

46. Kwon DH, Setser RM, Popovic ZB, et al. Association of myocardial fibrosis, electrocardiography and ventricular tachyarrhythmia in hypertrophic cardiomyopathy: a delayed contrast enhanced MRI study. Int J Cardiovasc Imaging 2008;24(6):617–25.

47. Rodriguez LM, Smeets JL, Timmermans C, et al. Radiofrequency catheter ablation of sustained monomorphic ventricular tachycardia in hypertrophic cardiomyopathy. J Cardiovasc Electrophysiol 1997; 8(7):803–6.

48. Lim KK, Maron BJ, Knight BP. Successful catheter ablation of hemodynamically unstable monomorphic ventricular tachycardia in a patient with hypertrophic cardiomyopathy and apical aneurysm. J Cardiovasc Electrophysiol 2009;20(4):445–7.

49. Inada K, Seiler J, Roberts-Thomson KC, et al. Substrate characterization and catheter ablation for monomorphic ventricular tachycardia in patients with apical hypertrophic cardiomyopathy. J Cardiovasc Electrophysiol 2011;22(1):41–8.

50. Santangeli P, Di Biase L, Lakkireddy D, et al. Radiofrequency catheter ablation of ventricular arrhythmias in patients with hypertrophic cardiomyopathy: safety and feasibility. Heart Rhythm 2010;7(8):1036–42.

51. Dukkipati SR, d'Avila A, Soejima K, et al. Long-term outcomes of combined epicardial and endocardial ablation of monomorphic ventricular tachycardia related to hypertrophic cardiomyopathy. Circ Arrhythm Electrophysiol 2011;4(2):185–94.

52. Nogami A. Mapping and ablating ventricular premature contractions that trigger ventricular fibrillation: trigger elimination and substrate modification. J Cardiovasc Electrophysiol 2015;26(1):110–5.

Sudden Cardiac Death Risk Stratification and the Role of the Implantable Cardiac Defibrillator

Sei Iwai, MD*

KEYWORDS

- Hypertrophic cardiomyopathy • Risk stratification • Sudden cardiac death • Syncope
- Ventricular fibrillation • Ventricular tachycardia

KEY POINTS

- Hypertrophic cardiomyopathy (HCM) is associated with an increased risk of sudden cardiac death (SCD).
- Given the heterogeneous nature of this disease entity, risk stratification of individuals with HCM remains challenging.
- Risk factors for SCD in HCM patients include history of ventricular fibrillation (VF), sustained ventricular tachycardia (VT), or SCD; family history of sudden death due to HCM; unexplained syncope; nonsustained VT; maximal left ventricular wall thickness over 3 cm; and abnormal blood pressure (BP) response during exercise.
- A newly developed HCM risk-SCD prediction model seems to more accurately assess risk of SCD in patients with HCM.
- Even though implantation of an implantable cardiac defibrillator (ICD) is effective in preventing SCD by terminating VT/VF in patients at increased risk, the importance of shared decision making cannot be understated.

Hypertrophic cardiomyopathy (HCM) is associated with an increased risk sudden cardiac death (SCD). HCM is also the most common cause of SCD in individuals less than 40 years of age.[1] Although the initial reported incidence of SCD was estimated to be as high as 6% per year, it was later appreciated that this was an overestimate due to referral bias of high-risk patients to tertiary-care centers.[2] Recent estimates have been in the range of approximately 1% per year or less.[3,4] The most common arrhythmia leading to SCD in HCM is ventricular fibrillation (VF). Asystole,[5] atrioventricular block,[6] accessory pathway conduction,[7] atrial fibrillation,[8]

and pulseless electrical activity have also been documented as contributing etiologies.

Risk stratification of patients with HCM remains a challenging task, partly due to the heterogeneous nature of the disease entity. Recent consensus statements and guidelines have attempted to address this issue to guide management.[9,10] This article aims to review the potential factors that contribute to the SCD risk in HCM and to discuss the role of the implantable cardiac defibrillator (ICD) in this population.

Traditional risk factors for SCD in HCM have included (1) prior personal history of VF, sustained

Disclosure Statement: Dr S. Iwai has received honoraria from Biosense-Webster, Biotronik, Boston Scientific, and Janssen Pharmaceuticals.
Cardiac Electrophysiology, New York Medical College, Westchester Medical Center Health System, Valhalla, NY, USA
* 19 Bradhurst Avenue, Suite 3850S, Hawthorne, NY 10532.
E-mail address: Sei.Iwai@wmchealth.org

Cardiol Clin 37 (2019) 63–72
https://doi.org/10.1016/j.ccl.2018.08.011
0733-8651/19/© 2018 Elsevier Inc. All rights reserved.

ventricular tachycardia (VT), or SCD; (2) family history of sudden death in a first-degree relative with HCM; (3) unexplained syncope; (4) nonsustained VT (NSVT); (5) maximal left ventricular (LV) wall thickness over 3 cm; and (6) abnormal blood pressure (BP) response during exercise (**Table 1**). The data for each of these clinical parameters as well as other factors that have been less well validated or have emerged more recently are reviewed.

PERSONAL HISTORY OF VENTRICULAR TACHYCARDIA/VENTRICULAR FIBRILLATION OR SUDDEN CARDIAC DEATH

Perhaps not surprising is that HCM patients with prior SCD or sustained VT are at high risk for recurrent episodes. Cecchi and colleagues[11] described the long-term outcome of 33 patients with HCM after resuscitated cardiac arrest. The event-free rate from recurrent cardiac arrest was 83%, 65%, and 53% at 1 year, 5 years, and 10 years, respectively. Subsequently, Elliott and colleagues[12] reported survival in a small series of 16 HCM patients with witnessed resuscitated VF or syncopal VT/VF when treated with low-dose amiodarone or ICDs. Eight patients were started on low-dose amiodarone and 6 underwent implantation of an ICD. The 5-year survival from death or ICD discharge was 59%.

FAMILY HISTORY OF SUDDEN CARDIAC DEATH

Although some studies have not demonstrated family history of SCD as a risk factor for SCD in multivariate analyses, other studies have supported the concept of family history being an independent predictor. Although definitions vary somewhat, a family history of SCD is usually considered significant if at least 1 first-degree relative has died suddenly before 40 years of age with or without a diagnosis of HCM or when SCD has occurred in a first-degree relative at any age with an established diagnosis of HCM. Bos and colleagues[13] investigated the rate of appropriate ICD interventions in 177 consecutive patients with HCM who had undergone ICD implantation for primary prevention of SCD based on the presence of at least 1 risk factor. Of the 177 patients, 91 (51%) had a family history of SCD in at least 1 first-degree relative. These 91 patients had a lower maximal LV wall thickness than the 86 patients without a family history of sudden death (21 ± 7 mm vs 25 ± 9 mm, respectively; $P = .04$). Furthermore, this was the only risk factor in 42 patients. Other risk factors used for ICD consideration in this study included (1) recent unexplained syncope, (2) abnormal BP response to treadmill exercise test, (3) massive LV hypertrophy (≥30 mm), and (4)

NSVT. During follow-up, 25 (14%) of the 177 patients experienced an appropriate ICD therapy, with the interval from ICD implantation to first appropriate ICD therapy 2.7 years. Of the 91 patients with family history of SCD, 13 (14%) had an appropriate ICD therapy compared with 12 (14%) of the 86 patients with no family history. Furthermore, the rate of ICD therapies was also similar between the groups with and without a family history of SCD (3.7/100 vs 3.1/100 person-years, respectively). When analyzing the group (42 patients) with family history as the only risk factor, 4 (10%) experienced an appropriate ICD therapy, with an event rate of 2.2/100 person-years. In comparison, 7 of the 50 patients (14%) with an ICD placed for reasons other than family history of SCD had an event rate of 3.4/100 person-years ($P = .2$).

UNEXPLAINED SYNCOPE

Syncope in HCM is common. Kofflard and colleagues[14] studied HCM patients in a large community-based population to identify risk factors for SCD and found that 43 of 225 patients (19%) had a history of syncope. Furthermore, syncope can have multiple etiologies, making diagnosis and management challenging. Besides sustained ventricular arrhythmias, possible mechanisms for syncope in HCM include arrhythmic etiologies, such as paroxysmal atrial fibrillation or SVT and complete heart block or sinus node dysfunction. Primary hemodynamic mechanisms include LV outflow tract (LVOT) obstruction, abnormal vascular control mechanisms and resultant inappropriate vasodilatation, and impaired filling due to preload reduction.[15] Syncope for which there is no underlying cause identified is associated with an increased risk of SCD.

The relationship between syncope and SCD was assessed in 1511 consecutive patients with HCM by Spirito and colleagues.[16] Syncope occurred in 205 patients (14%), including 153 (10%) with unexplained etiology and 52 (3%) with neurally mediated syncope. During a follow-up period of 5.6 years, the relative risk of SCD was 1.78 in patients with unexplained syncope and 0.91 in those with neurally mediated syncope compared with patients without syncope. In addition, patients with syncope within the prior 6 months had a hazard ratio (HR) of 4.89 compared with those with no syncope. Patients 40 years of age and older with remote (more than 5 years) episodes of syncope did not have an increased risk (HR 0.38) of SCD (**Fig. 1**).

The 2017 American College of Cardiology (ACC)/American Heart Association (AHA)/Heart Rhythm Society (HRS) syncope guideline statement[17] recommends that recent unexplained syncope be

Table 1
Clinical features associated with increased risk of sudden cardiac death in hypertrophic cardiomyopathy

Traditional Risk Factors	Other Risk Factors/ Modifiers
Prior personal history of VF, VT, or SCD	Maximal LVOT gradient >30 mm Hg
Family history of SCD and HCM	Myocardial fibrosis on CMR imaging
Unexplained syncope	LA diameter/size
NSVT	Specific genetic mutations
Maximal LV wall thickness over 3 cm	Younger age
Abnormal BP response to exercise	LV apical aneurysm

considered an independent predictor for SCD in HCM; thus, ICD implant is reasonable (class I indication). The recently published 2018 European Society of Cardiology (ESC) syncope guidelines[18] are consistent with this, recommending ICD implantation for HCM patients with syncope and other features indicative of high risk of SCD, utilizing the HCM risk-SCD model.[5]

NONSUSTAINED VENTRICULAR TACHYCARDIA

Although sustained VT is clearly associated with risk of SCD, NSVT has a somewhat lower predictive value. Despite this, Spirito and colleagues[19] followed 151 patients with no or mild heart failure symptoms, with no history of recurrent or recent syncope, who were not on cardiac medications, and who underwent ambulatory ECG monitoring. Of these patients, 42 had episodes of NSVT, ranging from 3 beats to 19 beats (35 [83%] had <10 beats), and 1 to 12 episodes in 24 hours (36 [86%] had <6 episodes). After a mean follow-up of 4.8 years, 6 died suddenly, 3 in the NSVT group and 3 in the group with no NSVT. The sudden death rate was 1.4% per year for the group with NSVT and 0.6% for those without (HR 2.4).

More recently, Monserrat and colleagues[20] reported their findings on 531 HCM patients assessed between 1988 and 2000 who underwent ambulatory ECG monitoring. During a mean follow-up of 70 months, 104 patients (19.6%) had NSVT on monitor. In patients 30 years of age or less, 5-year freedom from SCD was worse in those with NSVT (77.6% vs 94.1%, respectively). The odds ratio for SCD was 4.35 in this group, but only 2.16 (which did not reach statistical significance; $P = .1$) in

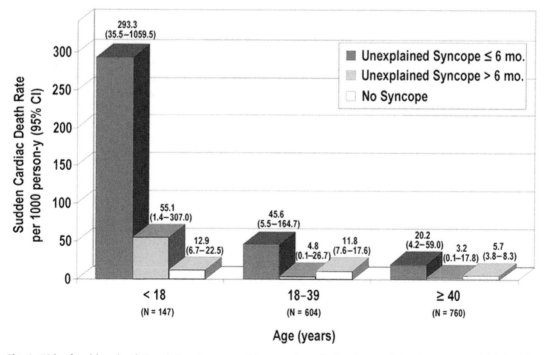

Fig. 1. Risk of sudden death in relation to age and temporal proximity of unexplained syncope to initial evaluation. Risk of sudden death was increased in all age groups with recent syncope (≤6 months). Conversely, risk of sudden death was not increased in adult patients (≥40 years old) with more distant syncopal events. (*From* Spirito P, Autore C, Rapezzi C, et al. Syncope and risk of sudden death in hypertrophic cardiomyopathy. Circulation 2009;119:1708; with permission.)

patients over age 30. Importantly, there was no relation between duration, frequency or rate of NSVT, and prognosis (**Fig. 2**).

Gimeno and colleagues[21] sought to determine the frequency of exercise-induced NSVT and its relation to SCD risk in 1380 patients referred to a cardiomyopathy clinic. During exercise, 24 patients had NSVT (13 had more than 1 run of NSVT), and 3 had VF. Exercise NSVT was associated with an increased risk of SCD (HR 2.82). Furthermore, patients with exercise NSVT/VF had more severe hypertrophy, larger left atria, and increased risk of SCD or ICD discharge (HR 3.73).

MAXIMAL LEFT VENTRICULAR WALL THICKNESS

Based on the hypothesis that more severe disease expression (ie, greater degree of LV wall thickening) correlates with worse outcomes, several studies have evaluated the relationship between the severity of LV hypertrophy and SCD in HCM. Most studies have shown an association (in univariate or multivariate analysis) between maximal LV wall thickness and SCD.

Olivotto and colleagues[22] analyzed the mortality rates of 237 patients with HCM, stratified by maximum LV thickness on echocardiogram into 5 groups. During a mean follow-up of 12 years, 36 patients died of cardiovascular causes, of which 16 were classified as SCD. Somewhat surprisingly, they found that maximum LV thickness did not seem associated with SCD risk or overall cardiovascular mortality. The distribution of SCD was not significantly different among the groups, except that the group with thickness values of 15 mm or less had a consistently benign clinical course. On the other extreme, in the group with LV thickness of 30 mm or greater, there was only 1 SCD event in patients diagnosed before age of 18 (17%) and none among 24 patients diagnosed at greater than or equal to 18 years of age.

Elliott and colleagues[23] reported that the risk of SCD associated with wall thickness of 30 mm or greater in patients without other risk factors is insufficient to justify aggressive prophylactic therapy and that because most sudden deaths occurred in patients with LV thickness less than 30 mm, the presence of mild hypertrophy could not be used to reassure patients that they had a good prognosis. They found that, in 630 consecutive patients, 39 died suddenly or had an appropriate ICD discharge. Even though they found a trend toward higher probability of SCD or ICD discharge with increasing wall thickness, only 10 of the 39 patients who had SCD had thicknesses of 30 mm or more. They contended that the number of additional risk factors was a better predictor of SCD risk.

Although data on the prognostic value of extreme LV thickness (30 mm or more) are somewhat mixed, there does seem to be some evidence pointing toward higher SCD risk with increasing thickness. Spirito and colleagues[24] assessed the relationship between LV thickness and mortality in 480 consecutive patients with HCM. Over a mean follow-up of 6.5 years, the risk of sudden death increased progressively and in direct relation to wall thickness. For example, the cumulative risk 20 years after initial evaluation was almost zero for patients with LV thickness under 20 mm but almost 40% in those 30 mm or thicker. The incidence rates per 1000 person-years was 0, 2.6, 7.4, 11.0, and 18.2 in patients with LV thicknesses of 15 mm or less, 16 mm to 19 mm, 20 mm to 24 mm, 25 mm to 29 mm,

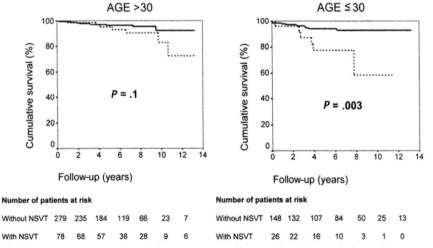

Fig. 2. Kaplan-Meier survival curves for sudden death in patients grouped by age (left panel: age>30, and right panel: age 30 and younger) with and without NSVT. Dotted lines = yes; solid lines = no. (*From* Monserrat L, Elliott PM, Gimeno JR, et al. Non-sustained ventricular tachycardia in hypertrophic cardiomyopathy: an independent marker of sudden death risk in young patients. J Am Coll Cardiol 2003;42:877; with permission.)

and 30 mm or greater, respectively. The highest rates were in the youngest patients; in those younger than 18 years of age at baseline, 5 died suddenly (incidence of SCD of 37.9 per 1000 person-years).

ABNORMAL BLOOD PRESSURE RESPONSE TO EXERCISE

Inappropriate systemic systolic BP response to exercise testing has been associated with higher risk of SCD. An abnormal response has been defined as failure to increase systolic BP by at least 20 mm Hg from rest to peak exercise or a fall of greater than 20 mm Hg from peak pressure. Sadoul and colleagues[25] prospectively studied consecutive young (age 8–40) HCM patients, using maximum symptom-limited treadmill exercise testing with continuous BP monitoring. Of the 161 patients studied, 60 (37%) had an abnormal response. There was no significant difference between the groups with normal and abnormal BP response with respect to recognized SCD risk factors, age, or gender. During a mean follow-up of 44 months, more patients in the group with abnormal response had SCD than in the group with normal response (15% vs 3%). Abnormal BP response had a 75% sensitivity, 66% specificity, 97% negative predictive value, and 15% positive predictive value for SCD.

OTHER POTENTIAL SUDDEN CARDIAC DEATH RISK FACTORS
Maximal Instantaneous Left Ventricular Outflow Tract Gradient

Although the data are somewhat conflicting, some studies have demonstrated higher SCD rates in patients with resting gradients over 30 mm Hg, a finding that is correlated with severity of LVOT obstruction. For example, Elliott and colleagues[26] reported that in a cohort of 917 patients with HCM, 288 had LVOT gradient at rest of over 30 mm Hg. During a median follow-up of 61 months, patients with an LVOT gradient had lower 5-year survival from all-cause death or cardiac transplantation (86.5% vs 90.1%). In addition, the magnitude of LVOT obstruction was associated with a higher rate of SCD or ICD discharges with relative risk of 1.36 per 20 mm Hg. In multivariate analysis, LVOT obstruction was an independent predictor of SCD/ICD discharges, with a 2.4-fold increase in risk. Other groups, however, including Efthimiadis and colleagues,[27] reported no difference in cumulative event-free survival from SCD between patients with and without LVOT gradient of 30 mm Hg or more, with a 92% survival rate in both groups after a mean follow-up of 32.4 months (see **Table 1**).

Myocardial Fibrosis on Cardiac Magnetic Resonance (CMR) Imaging

It has been postulated that myocardial fibrosis may represent myocardial tissue that can harbor ventricular tachyarrhythmias. Myocardial fibrosis, as seen by late gadolinium enhancement (LGE) on CMR imaging, has been associated with ventricular ectopy. Adabag and colleagues[28] studied the prevalence and frequency of ventricular arrhythmias (premature ventricular contractions [PVCs], couplets, and NSVT) on 24-hour Holter monitors and correlated them to LGE on CMR imaging in 177 HCM patients with either no or mild symptoms. Ventricular arrhythmias were more common in those with LGE compared with those without LGE (PVCs: 89% vs 72%; couplets: 40% vs 17%; and NSVT 28% vs 4%). Patients with LGE also had greater numbers of each type of ectopy. In addition, O'Hanlon and colleagues[29] were able to show an association between myocardial fibrosis and more clinically relevant endpoints. Specifically, they assessed the presence and amount of myocardial fibrosis in 217 consecutive HCM patients, of whom 136 (63%) showed fibrosis. Over a mean follow-up period of 3.1 years, 34 (25%) of the patients in the fibrosis group reached the combined primary endpoint of cardiovascular death, unplanned cardiovascular admission, sustained VF/VT, or appropriate ICD discharge, compared with only 6 (7.4%) of the patients without fibrosis (HR 3.4) (**Fig. 3**). In addition, overall risk increased with increasing extent of fibrosis (HR 1.16 per 5% increase).

More recently, Chan and colleagues[30] also assessed the relation between LGE and cardiovascular outcomes in 1293 HCM patients referred for CMR imaging. Patients were followed for a median of 3.3 years, and SCD events (including appropriate ICD interventions) occurred in 37 patients (3%). They demonstrated a continuous relationship between LGE (by percent LV mass) and SCD risk. Extent of LGE was associated with an increased risk of SCD with HR of 1.46 per 10% increase in LGE, even after adjusting for other relevant disease variables, and LGE of greater than or equal to 15% of LV mass was associated with a 2-fold increase in SCD risk, even in those patients otherwise considered at lower risk, with an event rate of 6% at 5 years. Furthermore, LGE also predicted development of end-stage HCM with systolic dysfunction (HR 1.80 per 10% increase in LGE).

Left Atrial Diameter

There has been a positive association reported between left atrial (LA) size and SCD. In an evaluation of syncope and risk of SCD in HCM, Spirito and colleagues[16] identified LA size (as well as age

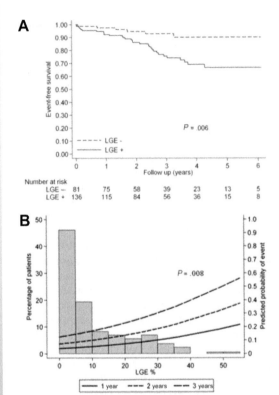

Fig. 3. (*A*) Fibrosis and development of primary endpoint. Kaplan-Meier unadjusted estimates of freedom from reaching combined primary endpoint (cardiovascular death, unplanned cardiovascular admission, sustained VT or VF, or appropriate implantable cardioverter-defibrillator discharge) in 217 HCM patients according the presence or absence of fibrosis. (*B*) Annual probability of primary endpoint correlating to amount of fibrosis. Predicted probability of reaching the combined primary endpoint at 1 year, 2 years, and 3 years on the basis of the overall percentage of fibrosis (*broken and unbroken lines*), plotted against the X axis on the right. The bar charts represent the overall percentage of patients with this amount of fibrosis, plotted on the X axis on the left. (*From* O'Hanlon R, Grasso A, Roughton M, et al. Prognostic significance of myocardial fibrosis in hypertrophic cardiomyopathy. J Am Coll Cardiol 2010;56:872; with permission.)

and LV wall thickness) in a set of multivariable Cox proportional hazard models as associated with SCD, with a relative risk of 1.03 (per millimeter as a continuous variable).

Genotype-Phenotype Associations

Comprehensive or targeted HCM genetic testing is recommended as a class I indication for any patient with a clinical diagnosis of HCM, based on clinical history, family history, and ECG and echocardiographic phenotype.[31] Mutation-specific genetic testing is recommended (also as a class I indication) for family members and appropriate

relatives after identification of the HCM-causative mutation in an index case. Currently, however, there is scant evidence to support the use of genetic testing to identify patients at high risk of SCD. Although SCD can occur in clusters in some families with HCM, initial studies reporting malignant sarcomere mutations were likely inaccurate. Subsequent studies in unselected populations demonstrated a lack of correlation with SCD events. Van Driest and colleagues[32] genotyped 293 unrelated HCM patients for 8 particular mutations that were considered benign defects and previously associated with near-normal survival. The investigators found the particular mutations to be rare (5 [1.7%] of 293 HCM patients). In addition, all 5 patients had undergone septal myectomies, and 3 of the 5 had a family history of SCD.

YOUNGER AGE

Some evidence points to younger age as a risk factor for SCD in HCM. McKenna and colleagues[33] reported on a retrospective analysis of 254 patients who were followed for a mean of 6 years, with 196 survivors, 32 who died of SCD and 26 who died from other causes. Young age (14 years or less) was one of the factors (along with syncope, severe dyspnea, family history of HCM and sudden death) that best predicted SCD. Age less than 30 years is included as a potential risk modifier for HCM patients in the recently published *2017 AHA/ACC/HRS Guideline for Management of Patients with Ventricular Arrhythmias and the Prevention of Sudden Cardiac Death*,[34] based on data from a multicenter retrospective registry,[1] and 1 prospective, single-center study.[35] Risk modifiers, when combined with a risk factor, potentially identify a patient with increased risk of SCD beyond the risk conveyed by the risk factor alone.

LEFT VENTRICULAR APICAL ANEURYSM

A small subset of patients with HCM, with prevalence of approximately 2%, develop an LV apical aneurysm.[36] These patients have worse prognosis, due to progressive heart failure as well as SCD. Based on limited data, these patients warrant consideration for strategies for SCD prevention.

ROLE OF IMPLANTABLE CARDIAC DEFIBRILLATOR IN PREVENTION OF SUDDEN CARDIAC DEATH IN HYPERTROPHIC CARDIOMYOPATHY

The indications for ICD implant in HCM follow the standard guidelines for treatment of arrhythmias in the general population,[34] with additional indications

Table 2
Indications for implantable cardiac defibrillator implant in hypertrophic cardiomyopathy

Risk Factor	2014 European Society of Cardiology Guidelines	2011 American College of Cardiology Foundation/American Heart Association Guidelines
History of SCD due to VT or VT	I	I
Sustained VT with syncope or hemodynamic compromise	I	I
5-y SCD risk estimate 6% or greater	IIa	
Family history of SCD caused by HCM		IIa
Maximal LV wall thickness of 30 mm or greater		IIa
Recent unexplained syncopal episode(s)		IIa
NSVT in presence of other SCD risk factors or modifiers		IIa
Abnormal BP response with exercise in presence of other SCD risk factors or modifiers		IIa
High-risk children with HCM (syncope, massive LV hypertrophy, family history of SCD)		IIa
5-y SCD risk estimate between 4% and 6%	IIb	
5-y SCD risk estimate <4% but with clinical features of proved prognostic importance	IIb	
NSVT without other SCD risk factors or modifiers		IIb
Abnormal BP response with exercise without other SCD risk factors or modifiers		IIb
5-y SCD risk estimate <4% with no other clinical features of proved prognostic importance	III	
HCM without an indication of increased risk		III
As a strategy to permit participation in competitive athletics		III
HCM with identified genotype in absence of clinical manifestations		III

Data from Gersh BJ, Maron BJ, Bonow RO, et al. 2011 ACCF/AHA guideline for the diagnosis and treatment of hypertrophic cardiomyopathy: a report of the American College of Cardiology Foundation/American Heart Association Task Force on Practice Guidelines. Circulation 2011:124:e783–831; and Elliott PM, Anastasakis A, Borger MA, et al. 2014 ESC Guidelines on diagnosis and management of hypertrophic cardiomyopathy. Eur Heart J 2014:35:2733–79.

based on the presence of the risk factors discussed previously. Although these clinical risk factors are associated with an increased relative risk of SCD, the positive predictive value of any individual factor is low, given the relatively low frequency of SCD.

Prophylactic treatment with an ICD is the standard of care for patients with HCM who are believed at high risk of SCD, albeit this is based on limited data from observational studies. For example, in a multicenter registry study of ICDs (implanted between 1986 and 2003) in 506 unrelated patients with HCM, ICDs were found effective in terminating VT or VF.[37] These patients were deemed to be at high risk for sudden death due to presence of traditional risk factors. ICD interventions terminated VT/VF in 103 patients (20%), with intervention rates of 10.6% and 3.6% per year for secondary and primary prevention, respectively.

O'Mahony and colleagues[38] used data from a multicenter, retrospective, longitudinal cohort study of 3675 patients and developed and validated a new SCD risk prediction model (HCM risk-SCD). The study cohort consisted of consecutively evaluated patients with HCM followed at 6 European centers. Patients that were more than 16 years of age, without prior VF or sustained VT, and without metabolic diseases or syndromic causes of HCM were included. The risk of SCD in 5 years is estimated using the following equation:

$$\text{Probability}_{\text{SCD at 5 y}} = 1 - 0.998^{\exp(\text{prognostic index})}$$

where *prognostic index* = [0.15939858 × maximal wall thickness (mm)] − [0.00294271 × maximal wall thickness^2 (mm^2)] + [0.0259082 × LA diameter (mm)] + [0.00446131 × maximal (rest/Valsalva) LVOT gradient (mm Hg)] + [0.4583082 × family history SCD] + [0.82639195 × NSVT] + [0.71650361 × unexplained syncope] − [0.01 799934 × age at clinical evaluation (years)]. In a head-to-head comparison with a model using 4 major risk factors, the performance of this prediction model was substantially better.

In a recent study that sought to externally validate the HCM risk-SCD prediction model in a geographically diverse cohort (from the United States, Europe, the Middle East, and Asia), O'Mahony and colleagues[39] included 3703 patients, of whom 73 (2%) had SCD within 5 years of follow-up. The validation study revealed a calibration slope of 1.02, C-index of 0.70, and D-statistic of 1.17. In a complete case analysis, patients with a predicted 5-year risk of less than 4% had an observed incidence of 1.4%, and patients with a predicted risk of greater than or equal to 6% had an observed incidence of 8.9%. Importantly, for every 13 patients with an estimated 5-year SCD risk of greater than or equal to 6% in whom an ICD is implanted, 1 patient can be potentially saved from SCD; that is, the number needed to treat to save 1 life is 13. This number needed to treat is approximately equivalent to the results from the Sudden Cardiac Death in Heart Failure Trial,[40] which plays an important role in the indications for ICD implant for primary prevention of SCD in patients with ischemic and nonischemic cardiomyopathy.

Even with these clinical data, selection of patients with HCM who are appropriate for ICD implantation for primary prevention of SCD can be challenging from medical and emotional standpoints. Many of the patients are young, and it is essential to discuss the potential ICD-related complications with the patient (and often the patient's family). Lin and colleagues[41] described the complications associated with ICD implantation in 181 HCM patients who were followed for a mean of 59 ± 42 months. Although the time period for inclusion (1988–2005) included ICDs implanted via thoracotomy (prior to 1994), the data highlight some of the potential issues with ICDs in the HCM population. The mean age was 44 ± 17 years (27% were <35 years), with 62% male patients and 86% having ICDs for primary prevention; 108 patients (60%) had a dual-chamber device implanted and 65 patients (36%) had a total of 88 complications, including 42 patients (33%) who had inappropriate ICD shocks. Although current modern programming of ICDs with longer detection times and/or high detection rates have been shown to decrease the frequency of inappropriate ICD therapies (and improve mortality),[42] the devices in this trial were programmed fairly judiciously, with a VF zone with cycle length cutoff of less than 220 ms and therapies for VT generally not used. Complication rates were highest in the first year postimplant (19%); 47 device implant–related complications occurred (26%), including pocket hematoma, acute upper extremity deep vein thrombosis, pneumothorax, lead revision, device infection, and high defibrillation thresholds. Although complication rates with current ICD systems might be expected to be somewhat lower, they are still not insignificant. Kirkfeldt and colleagues[43] reported data from a Danish registry of 562 patients, with 9.5% experiencing at least 1 complication. Similarly, in an Ontario ICD registry of 3340 patients, 172 patients (7.4%) with ICDs implanted for primary prevention and 76 (7.6%) for secondary prevention experienced a complication, including major complications in 3.8% and 4.8%, respectively.[44]

The 2014 ESC guidelines[10] for diagnosis and treatment of HCM recommend ICD implantation in the following patients, assuming a life expectancy of over 1 year: (1) those who have survived a cardiac arrest due to VT or VF or who have spontaneous sustained VT causing syncope or hemodynamic compromise (class I indication); (2) those with an estimated 5-year risk of sudden death of greater than or equal to 6% as per the HCM risk-SCD prediction model, after a detailed clinical assessment (class IIa indication); (3) those with an estimated 5-year risk of SCD between 4% and 6%, after detailed clinical assessment (class IIb indication); and (4) those with an estimated 5-year risk of SCD of less than 4% only when they have clinical features that are of proved prognostic importance. ICD implantation is not recommended in patients with an estimated 5-year risk of SCD of less than 4% and no other clinical features that are of proved prognostic importance (**Table 2**).

The 2011 ACC Foundation/AHA guidelines[9] for diagnosis and treatment of HCM recommend comprehensive SCD risk stratification to determine presence of any of the following: (1) personal history of VF, sustained VT, or SCD event; (2) family history of SCD; (3) unexplained syncope; (4) documented NSVT on Holter monitoring; and (5) maximal LV wall thickness of 30 mm or greater. In addition, other clinical risk factors can be considered. Regarding ICD implantation, these guidelines stress the importance of shared decision making. ICD implant is recommended for (1) patients with prior cardiac arrest, VF, or hemodynamically significant VT (class I indication); (2) patients with family history (first-degree relative) of SCD caused by HCM, maximal LV wall thickness of greater than or equal to 30 mm, or 1 or more recent and unexplained syncopal episodes (class IIa indication); (3) patients with NSVT (especially if <30 years of age) in presence of other SCD risk factors/modifiers (class IIa); (4) those with an abnormal BP response to exercise in the presence of other SCD risk factors/modifiers; and (5) high-risk children with HCM (based on unexplained syncope, massive LV hypertrophy, or family history of SCD) after considering the high complication rate of long-term ICD implantation (class IIa) (see **Table 2**).

SUMMARY

HCM is associated with an increased risk of sudden death, although perhaps not as significantly as previously believed. Given the heterogeneous nature of this disease entity, risk stratification of individuals with HCM remains challenging. The recent HCM risk-SCD prediction model[38] seems to perform well in assessing individual SCD risk. Even though ICDs are effective in preventing SCD by terminating VT/VF in patients at increased risk, the importance of shared decision making in deciding whether or not to undergo ICD implantation cannot be understated.

REFERENCES

1. Maron BJ, Shen W-K, Link MS, et al. Efficacy of implantable cardioverter-defibrillators for the prevention of sudden death in patients with hypertrophic cardiomyopathy. N Engl J Med 2000;342:365–73.

2. Maron BJ, Spirito P. Impact of patient selection biases on the perception of hypertrophic cardiomyopathy and its natural history. Am J Cardiol 1993;72:970–2.

3. Elliot PM, Gimeno JR, Thaman R, et al. Historical trends in reported survival rates in patients with hypertrophic cardiomyopathy. Heart 2006;92:785–91.

4. Maron BJ, Olivotto I, Spirito P, et al. Epidemiology of hypertrophic cardiomyopathy-related death: revisited in a large non-referral-based patient population. Circulation 2000;102:858–64.

5. Joseph S, Balcon R, McDonald L. Syncope in hypertrophic obstructive cardiomyopathy due to asystole. Br Heart J 1972;34:974–6.

6. Barriales-Villa R, Centurion-Inda R, Fernandez-Fernandez X, et al. Severe cardiac conduction disturbances and pacemaker implantation in patients with hypertrophic cardiomyopathy. Rev Esp Cardiol 2010;63:985–8.

7. Krikler DM, Davies MJ, Rowland E, et al. Sudden death in hypertrophic cardiomyopathy: associated accessory atrioventricular pathways. Br Heart J 1980;43:245–51.

8. Stafford WJ, Trohman RG, Bilsker M, et al. Cardiac arrest in an adolescent with atrial fibrillation and hypertrophic cardiomyopathy. J Am Coll Cardiol 1986;7:701–4.

9. Gersh BJ, Maron BJ, Bonow RO, et al. 2011 ACCF/AHA guideline for the diagnosis and treatment of hypertrophic cardiomyopathy: a report of the American College of Cardiology Foundation/American Heart Association task force on practice guidelines. Circulation 2011;124:e783–831.

10. Elliott PM, Anastasakis A, Borger MA, et al. 2014 ESC guidelines on diagnosis and management of hypertrophic cardiomyopathy. Eur Heart J 2014;35:2733–79.

11. Cecchi F, Maron BJ, Epstein SE. Long-term outcome of patients with hypertrophic cardiomyopathy successfully resuscitated after cardiac arrest. J Am Coll Cardiol 1989;13:1283–8.

12. Elliott PM, Sharma S, Varnava A, et al. Survival after cardiac arrest or sustained ventricular tachycardia in patients with hypertrophic cardiomyopathy. J Am Coll Cardiol 1999;33:1596–601.

13. Bos JM, Maron BJ, Ackerman MJ, et al. Role of family history of sudden death in risk stratification and prevention of sudden death with implantable defibrillators in hypertrophic cardiomyopathy. Am J Cardiol 2010;106:1481–6.

14. Kofflard MJM, Cate FJT, van der Lee C, et al. Hypertrophic cardiomyopathy in a large community-based population: clinical outcome and identification of risk factors for sudden cardiac death and clinical deterioration. J Am Coll Cardiol 2003;41:987–93.

15. Williams L, Frenneaux M. Syncope in hypertrophic cardiomyopathy: mechanisms and consequences for treatment. Europace 2007;9:817–22.

16. Spirito P, Autore C, Rapezzi C, et al. Syncope and risk of sudden death in hypertrophic cardiomyopathy. Circulation 2009;119:1703–10.

17. Shen W-K, Sheldon RS, Benditt DG, et al. 2017 ACC/AHA/HRS guideline for the evaluation and management of patients with syncope. Heart Rhythm 2017;14(8):e155–217.

18. Brignole M, Moya A, deLange FJ, et al. 2018 ESC guidelines for the diagnosis and management of syncope. Eur Heart J 2018;39:1883–948.

19. Spirito P, Rapezzi C, Autore C, et al. Prognosis of asymptomatic patients with hypertrophic cardiomyopathy and nonsustained ventricular tachycardia. Circulation 1994;90:2743–7.

20. Monserrat L, Elliott PM, Gimeno JR, et al. Non-sustained ventricular tachycardia in hypertrophic cardiomyopathy: an independent marker of sudden death risk in young patients. J Am Coll Cardiol 2003;42:873–9.

21. Gimeno JR, Tomé-Esteban M, Lofiego C, et al. Exercise-induced ventricular arrhythmias and risk of sudden cardiac death in patients with hypertrophic cardiomyopathy. Eur Heart J 2009;30:2599–605.

22. Olivotto I, Gistri R, Petrone P, et al. Maximum left ventricular thickness and risk of sudden death in patients with hypertrophic cardiomyopathy. J Am Coll Cardiol 2003;41:315–21.

23. Elliott PM, Gimeno Blanes JR, Mahon NG, et al. Relation between severity of left-ventricular hypertrophy and prognosis in patients with hypertrophic cardiomyopathy. Lancet 2001;357:420–4.

24. Spirito P, Bellone P, Harris KM, et al. Magnitude of left ventricular hypertrophy and risk of sudden death in hypertrophic cardiomyopathy. N Engl J Med 2000; 342:1778–85.

25. Sadoul N, Prasad K, Elliott PM, et al. Prospective prognostic assessment of blood pressure response during exercise in patients with hypertrophic cardiomyopathy. Circulation 1997;96:2987–91.

26. Elliott PM, Gimeno JR, Tomé MT, et al. Left ventricular outflow tract obstruction and sudden death risk in patients with hypertrophic cardiomyopathy. Eur Heart J 2006;27:1933–41.

27. Efthimiadis GK, Parcharidou DG, Giannakoulas G, et al. Left ventricular outflow tract obstruction as a risk factor for sudden cardiac death in hypertrophic cardiomyopathy. Am J Cardiol 2009;104:695–9.

28. Adabag AS, Maron BJ, Appelbaum E, et al. Occurrence and frequency of arrhythmias in hypertrophic cardiomyopathy in relation to delayed enhancement on cardiovascular magnetic resonance. J Am Coll Cardiol 2008;51:1369–74.

29. O'Hanlon R, Grasso A, Roughton M, et al. Prognostic significance of myocardial fibrosis in hypertrophic cardiomyopathy. J Am Coll Cardiol 2010;56:867–74.

30. Chan RH, Maron BJ, Olivotto I, et al. Prognostic value of quantitative contrast-enhanced cardiovascular magnetic resonance for the evaluation of sudden death risk in patients with hypertrophic cardiomyopathy. Circulation 2014;130(6):484–95.

31. Ackerman MJ, Priori SG, Willems S, et al. HRS/EHRA expert consensus statement on the state of genetic testing for the channelopathies and cardiomyopathies. Heart Rhythm 2011;8:1308–39.

32. Van Driest SL, Ackerman MJ, Ommen SR, et al. Prevalence and severity of "benign" mutations in the β-myosin heavy chain, cardiac troponin T, and α-tropomyosin genes in hypertrophic cardiomyopathy. Circulation 2002;106:3085–90.

33. McKenna W, Deanfield J, Faruqui A, et al. Prognosis in hypertrophic cardiomyopathy: role of age and clinical, electrocardiographic and hemodynamic features. Am J Cardiol 1981;479(3):532–8.

34. Al-Khatib SM, Stevenson WG, Ackerman MJ, et al. 2017 AHA/ACC/HRS guideline for management of patients with ventricular arrhythmias and the prevention of sudden cardiac death. Heart Rhythm 2017. https://doi.org/10.1016/j.hrthm.2017.10.036.

35. Maki S, Ikeda H, Muro A, et al. Predictors of sudden cardiac death in hypertrophic cardiomyopathy. Am J Cardiol 1998;82:774–8.

36. Maron MS, Finely JJ, Bos JM, et al. Prevalence, clinical significance, and natural history of left ventricular apical aneurysms in hypertrophic cardiomyopathy. Circulation 2008;118(15):1541–9.

37. Maron BJ, Spirito P, Shen W-K. Implantable cardioverter-defibrillators and prevention of sudden cardiac death in hypertrophic cardiomyopathy. JAMA 2007;298(4):405–12.

38. O'Mahony C, Jichi F, Pavlou M, et al. A novel clinical risk prediction model for sudden cardiac death in hypertrophic cardiomyopathy (HCM Risk-SCD). Eur Heart J 2014;35:2010–20.

39. O'Mahony C, Jichi F, Ommen SR, et al. An international external validation study of the 2014 European Society of Cardiology guideline on sudden cardiac death prevention in hypertrophic cardiomyopathy (Evidence from HCM). Circulation 2018;137:1015–23.

40. Bardy GH, Lee KL, Mark DB, et al. Amiodarone or an implantable cardioverter-defibrillator for congestive heart failure. N Engl J Med 2005;352:225–37.

41. Lin G, Nishimura RA, Gersh BJ, et al. Device complications and inappropriate implantable cardioverter defibrillator shocks in patients with hypertrophic cardiomyopathy. Heart 2009;95(9):709–14.

42. Moss AJ, Schuger C, Beck CA, et al. Reduction in inappropriate therapy and mortality through ICD programming. N Engl J Med 2012;367(24):2275–83.

43. Kirkfeldt RE, Johansen JB, Nohr EA, et al. Complications after cardiac implantable electronic device implantations: an analysis of a complete, nationwide cohort in Denmark. Eur Heart J 2014;35:1186–94.

44. Lee DS, Krahn AD, Healey JS, et al. Evaluation of early complications related to de novo cardioverter defibrillator implantation. J Am Coll Cardiol 2010;55:774–82.

Role of Advanced Testing
Invasive Hemodynamics, Endomyocardial Biopsy, and Cardiopulmonary Exercise Testing

Gregg M. Lanier, MD[a],*, John T. Fallon, MD, PhD[b],
Srihari S. Naidu, MD[c]

KEYWORDS

- Hypertrophic cardiomyopathy • Hemodynamic assessment • Cardiac catheterization
- Endomyocardial biopsy • Cardiopulmonary exercise testing • Restrictive heart failure

KEY POINTS

- Invasive testing with cardiac catheterization provides hemodynamic data to guide the treatment of hypertrophic cardiomyopathy, identifies patients who might benefit from septal reduction therapy, and assesses for other comorbidities that may be contributing to symptoms.
- Endomyocardial biopsy has no routine role in the evaluation of hypertrophic cardiomyopathy, except in cases where other conditions are being considered.
- Cardiopulmonary exercise testing provides an objective assessment of functional capacity in hypertrophic cardiomyopathy.
- A peak oxygen consumption (Vo_2) of less than 14 mL/kg/min (or <50% predicted for age) and a VE/VCO_2 slope of greater than 35 indicate a poor prognosis and possible benefit from referral for heart transplantation.

INTRODUCTION

Patients with hypertrophic cardiomyopathy (HCM) have complex manifestations of not only their cardiac disease, but often from other disease states that modify the clinical presentation.[1] Accordingly, the phenotype and relevant consequences may need to be confirmed or refuted invasively, adding clarity to the diagnosis and allowing for a determination of other nonrelated conditions. Therefore, in a subset of patients, various invasive or supplemental diagnostic testing may be required. This review focuses on the role of invasive hemodynamic evaluation in HCM. In addition, although rarely needed, the role of endomyocardial biopsy will be reviewed, as well as characteristic histologic findings of this disease. And finally, the role of cardiopulmonary exercise testing (CPET) is discussed, including when this modality is required or helpful, how to interpret the data, and how it can be used to guide treatment decisions or evaluate the effects of invasive or drug

Disclosure Statement: The authors have no relevant financial relationships.
[a] Pulmonary Hypertension Program, Heart Failure, Westchester Medical Center, New York Medical College, 100 Woods Road, Macy Pavilion Room 110, Valhalla, NY 10595, USA; [b] Department of Clinical Laboratories and Pathology, Westchester Medical Center, New York Medical College, 100 Woods Road, Macy Pavilion Room 106, Valhalla, NY 10595, USA; [c] Hypertrophic Cardiomyopathy Program, Cardiac Catheterization Laboratory, Westchester Medical Center, New York Medical College, 100 Woods Road, Macy Pavilion Room 106, Valhalla, NY 10595, USA
* Corresponding author.
E-mail address: Gregg.lanier@wmchealth.org

Cardiol Clin 37 (2019) 73–82
https://doi.org/10.1016/j.ccl.2018.08.010

therapies. Together, this review highlights the complexity of this disease and the depths of evaluation that are required to provide comprehensive, high-quality, and individualized care.

INVASIVE HEMODYNAMICS

Patients with HCM may have a myriad of signs and symptoms, including dyspnea, fatigue, wheezing, lower extremity edema, chest pain, palpitations, lightheadedness, or syncope. Dyspnea and shortness of breath may occur from reduced cardiac output with forward heart failure (HF), pulmonary vascular congestion from backward HF, or from elevated pulmonary vascular resistance (PVR) either from longstanding HCM or primary pulmonary pathology. Edema may be cardiogenic from elevated right-sided pressures from right HF or secondary to total body volume overload, varicose veins, or deep vein thrombosis. Chest pain may develop from elevated end-diastolic pressure, systemic hypertension, reduced coronary perfusion from arteriopathy, or from epicardial coronary artery disease. Dizziness and syncope may result from arrhythmias, left ventricular obstructive physiology, or the inability to augment cardiac output appropriately to match decreases in systemic vascular resistance with exercise. Finally, wheezing may be a manifestation of pulmonary congestion or from pulmonary disease such as asthma. Therefore, given all these potential conditions that could confound the symptoms of a patient with HCM, right and left heart catheterization provides objective hemodynamic information to further understand the patient's physiology and rule in or out other comorbidities. Indications for cardiac catheterization in HCM are listed in **Box 1**.

Performance of the right heart catheterization begins with measuring the right atrial pressure.[2] All pressures should be end-expiratory, especially in those with significant respiratory variation, such as patients with obesity or lung disease. Right atrial pressure of greater than 8 to 10 mm Hg indicates significant systemic congestion and/or right ventricular (RV) failure, and may result in lower extremity edema. RV pressure may reflect pulmonary pressures, but may also be a manifestation of RV outflow tract obstruction, especially in young patients with massive septal hypertrophy. Advancement of the catheter from RV to PA will elucidate this gradient. In general, owing to the low pressure system, mild to moderate gradients can be largely ignored, whereas severe gradients of greater than 30 to 50 mm Hg are notable and should be considered contributory. Pulmonary hypertension is graded mild (mean pulmonary artery pressure

---

> **Box 1**
> **Indications for cardiac catheterization in hypertrophic cardiomyopathy**
>
> Evaluation of symptoms
>
> Evaluation of coronary disease
>
> Preprocedure planning for alcohol septal ablation
>
> Determination of resting or latent obstruction
>
> Localization of obstruction
>
> Evaluation of pulmonary hypertension
>
> Evaluation of volume status
>
> Evaluation of cardiac output and index

25–35 mm Hg), moderate (35–45 mm Hg), or severe (>45 mm Hg), and a calculation of the transpulmonary gradient and PVR are useful markers of secondary or intrinsic pulmonary disease. Although PVR values of less than 3 Wood units are likely not significantly contributory to the clinical picture, those greater than 3 Wood units, and certainly those greater than 5 Wood units, should be addressed by formal pulmonary and/or pulmonary hypertension consultation. The pulmonary capillary wedge pressure is important to determine the volume status, as well as the transpulmonary gradient and PVR. Pulmonary capillary wedge pressures in patients with HCM usually are slightly greater than in normal individuals, and determined by their level of diastolic dysfunction. Indeed, values of 12 to 15 mm Hg are expected and likely needed to produce appropriate cardiac output and to decrease the chances of preload-dependent obstruction. Therefore, values lower than this range often require hydration, whereas higher values require various levels of diuretics, starting with the most mild forms. For values of greater than 20 to 25 mm Hg, loop diuretics may be needed to alleviate symptoms, even in obstructive patients.

The cardiac output and index can be calculated by Fick or thermodilution techniques. Owing to the limitations of each, it is recommended that both are determined in these patients to get a better sense of the range of output. Low outputs are typical in patients with HCM owing to diastolic dysfunction (both myocardial and owing to cavity obliteration), obstruction (a form of systolic dysfunction), and secondary features such as systolic anterior motion of the mitral valve-related mitral regurgitation (which further limits stroke volume), atrial fibrillation, and an increased PVR. It is important that the cardiac output be determined to understand the relative contributions of each of these to the drop in output. For example, if the PVR seems to be the rate-limiting step, then the focus should be on that abnormality. If, in contrast, the diastolic dysfunction is the rate-limiting step, then the focus should be there. And if the glaring pathophysiologic component is the obstruction to flow, then invasive therapies are needed and likely to be beneficial.

Accordingly, a critical area to master is the elucidation of obstructive physiology, and determination of its magnitude, because the elimination of obstruction can improve stroke volume initially through more complete ejection and the decrease in systolic anterior motion of the mitral valve-related mitral regurgitation, and over time through remodeling that improves diastolic function. Two transducers are required to measure and compare pressures and calculate gradients.[2,3] Usually, a pigtail catheter is placed at the LV apex, and a second catheter is placed in the ascending aorta. Any resting gradient in the patient without aortic stenosis is attributed to resting outflow tract or midcavity obstruction. Provocative maneuvers are then performed. These maneuvers should include the strain phase of the Valsalva maneuver alone, induction of a premature ventricular contraction to reveal the Brockenbrough-Braunwauld-Morrow sign,

and with the provocation of a premature ventricular contraction after 10 to 15 seconds of the strain phase of the Valsalva maneuver. The aortic tracing in the patient with dynamic obstruction will evidence a spike and dome waveform, indicative of early rapid ejection before obstruction, the cessation of flow during obstruction, and a slow later ejection as obstruction is relieved but ventricular pressure remains above aortic pressure. During worsening obstruction by Valsalva or Brockenbrough, the gradient increases, and the spike and dome configuration becomes more evident. The Brockenbrough-Braunwal-Morrow sign is characterized by a decrease in the pulse pressure in the ventricular beat after the premature ventricular contraction (**Fig. 1**). This decrease in pulse pressure indicates a decreased stroke volume from worsening obstruction, which also results in a larger gradient on this beat and a more marked spike and dome aortic tracing. Gradients of greater than 30 mm Hg indicate obstructive disease, whereas those of greater than 50 mm Hg indicate candidacy for septal reduction therapy, based on national guidelines.

A key part of the hemodynamic assessment is localizing the level of obstruction. Accordingly, the LV pigtail catheter can be exchanged for an

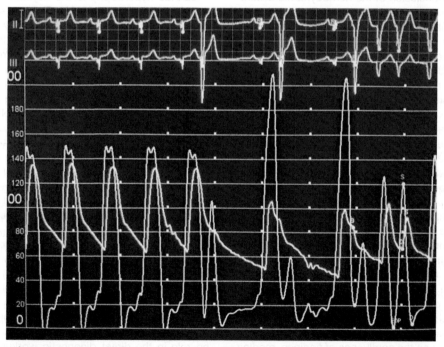

Fig. 1. Hemodynamic tracings of left ventricular (*orange*) and aortic (*blue*) pressures showing a resting gradient followed by induction of a premature ventricular contraction (PVC), which elicits a decrease in the pulse pressure of the next beat and an increase in the gradient. The decrease in pulse pressure signifies a decrease in stroke volume owing to obstruction. Note the spike and dome configuration of the aortic tracing in the post-PVC beat, a classic hemodynamic sign in obstructive hypertrophic cardiomyopathy.

end-hole catheter and gradual pullback can determine the precise location of obstruction, as well as rule out concomitant aortic valvular stenosis. If aortic stenosis is present, the valvular gradient can be isolated by placing the end-hole catheter above the muscular obstruction and below the aortic valve. At this level, there should be no provokable gradient, and the mean gradient across the valve can be used to calculate a valve area. The relative contributions of the aortic mean gradient can be compared with any subvalvular mean gradient and any provokable gradient can be attributed to the subvalvular obstruction. In this manner, the relative contributions of aortic valvular and subvalvular obstructions can be determined, leading to decisions regarding invasive therapies on 1 or both anatomic impediments to flow.[4]

In some centers, transeptal catheterization is performed to place a pigtail catheter consistently below the outflow tract (mitral inflow area) for more precise measurements.[2] Using a combination of retrograde and transeptal approaches, it is possible to elucidate midcavity, outflow tract and valvular obstructions coexisting in 1 patient. However, owing to some risk of transeptal puncture, this approach is not routine and used only in select cases.

At the conclusion of the hemodynamic assessment, an LV-gram is typically performed through the pigtail catheter. In many cases, this assessment can reveal apical HCM and/or the presence of apical aneurysm. In addition, it may determine that the pigtail never reached the true apex and thereby underestimated any midventricular gradients. Advancement of the pigtail catheter to the true apex will result in more accurate gradient assessments.

After performing a right and left heart catheterization in a patient with HCM, the clinician will better understand the contributions of congestion and volume overload, PVR, and obstruction to any reduction in cardiac output. Decreased cardiac output without derangements in these variables usually is due to diastolic dysfunction or other intrinsic or related valvular disease such as mitral regurgitation or secondary to arrhythmias such as atrial fibrillation. Coronary angiography performed at the end of the study is useful to exclude coronary disease as a contributor and for assessment of the coronary perforator artery anatomy if alcohol septal ablation is being considered. Depending on the confluence of findings, medications may be changed (such as beta-blockers, disopyramide, or diuretics), and invasive therapies may be contemplated, including surgical myectomy, alcohol septal ablation, or heart transplantation. In this manner, the invasive assessment is a powerful tool in understanding and individualizing each patient's physiology.

ENDOMYOCARDIAL BIOPSY

The gross and histologic features of HCM, including ventricular and myocyte hypertrophy, myocyte disarray, and interstitial/endocardial fibrosis, first described by Teare in 1958,[5] are the consequence of underlying sarcomeric gene mutation(s) plus environmental factors that produce the clinical manifestations of HCM, including subaortic stenosis, mitral regurgitation, HF, arrhythmias, and sudden death.[6]

HCM is an autosomal-dominant genetic disease, but the sarcomere mutation(s) are pleiotropic (when 1 gene influences ≥ 2 seemingly unrelated phenotypic traits). Accordingly, mutation(s) in the same gene may manifest as different forms of HCM, namely, dilated cardiomyopathy, restrictive cardiomyopathy, and even left ventricular noncompaction syndrome.[7] Even pathologically, patients with HCM may exhibit a variable phenotype with ventricular hypertrophy being the cardinal gross manifestation, whereas myocyte hypertrophy, myocyte disarray, and interstitial fibrosis are key histopathologic hallmarks.

Cardiac hypertrophy is the keystone to gross pathologic diagnosis of HCM. The hypertrophy is frequently asymmetrical, predominantly involving the basal interventricular septum just below the aortic valve, but may be concentric or involve only the apical septum. In HCM (aka, asymmetrical septal hypertrophy), the ratio of the thickness of the septum to the free wall of the ventricle is greater than or equal to 1.3/1.0. Nonobstructive HCM may present with concentric hypertrophy but, very rarely, only the inferior or lateral walls are the sites of hypertrophy. Other frequent gross pathologic features include elongation and fibrosis of the anterior leaflet of the mitral valve, myxoid degeneration of the posterior mitral valve leaflet, and abnormal insertion of the associated papillary muscle[8] (**Fig. 2**). Endocardial fibrosis is also a common finding in obstructive HCM and appears on the basal septum as a mirror image of the anterior leaflet of the mitral valve (see **Fig. 2B**). The right ventricle is seldom involved by hypertrophy in patients with HCM and only rarely manifests outflow tract obstruction owing to infundibular wall hypertrophy. RV endomyocardial biopsy plays no role in the direct diagnostic workup of HCM except to rule out conditions that may mimic HCM such as amyloidosis, Fabry's disease, and other metabolic storage diseases. In the current era, this evaluation may become necessary in

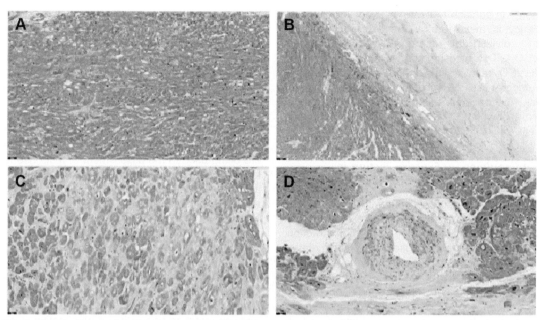

Fig. 2. Photomicrograph of septectomy specimen from patient with obstructive hypertrophic cardiomyopathy showing myocyte hypertrophy and disarray (*A*) (hematoxylin-eosin, original magnification ×100), endocardial fibrosis (*B*) (hematoxylin-eosin, original magnification ×200), interstitial fibrosis (*C*) (hematoxylin-eosin, original magnification ×50), dysplastic intramural coronary artery (*D*) (hematoxylin-eosin, original magnification ×50).

select cases, especially in the young and in those in whom genetic testing or noncardiac disease suggests an alternate diagnosis.

Histologically in HCM, the cardiac myocytes are enlarged with outsized, pleiotropic nuclei. The myocytes have a disarrayed pattern, with a loss of normal parallel alignment and rather haphazard orientation, which often presents a swirling appearance to the mural architecture (see **Fig. 2**A). This myocyte disarray typically involves only the midmural regions of the hypertrophied interventricular septum in obstructive and apical HCM, but is often present midmurally and circumferentially or in the free walls of the left ventricle in nonobstructive forms of HCM. This pattern of myocyte disarray is also present in normal hearts at the anterior and inferior junctions of the right and left ventricular walls.

Multifocal interstitial fibrosis is a common feature that may contribute to the restrictive physiology often found in HCM (see **Fig. 2**C). The intramural coronary arteries regularly exhibit a dysplastic appearance with irregular wall thickening and narrowed lumina. These arteries are imbedded in the interstitial fibrous tissue and this pathology may contribute to myocardial ischemia seen in certain patients with HCM (see **Fig. 2**D).

The histopathologic features are often appreciated in septal myectomy specimens obtained at the time of surgical myectomy for the treatment

of obstructive HCM. However, a recent report suggests that the microscopic findings in septectomy specimens from patients with obstructive HCM, membranous subaortic stenosis, and secondary subaortic stenosis owing to calcific valvular aortic stenosis show no significant differences.[9]

CARDIOPULMONARY EXERCISE TESTING

There are several ways to objectively measure functional capacity. A patient's ability to exercise, as measured by either treadmill or bicycle ergometry, has been validated extensively in estimating prognosis and risk in coronary artery disease.[10] Workload achieved, estimated as metabolic equivalents, is another valuable result of exercise testing, and has been shown to predict mortality in HF.[11] Heart rate and blood pressure changes during exercise can document chronotropic incompetence and abnormal blood pressure response with increased workload. Adding to these findings, CPET provides additional objective information that can offer insight into a patient's cardiac and pulmonary limitations to exercise. A mouth piece with a nonrebreathing valve and a metabolic cart are used during exercise to analyze breath-by-breath percent O_2 and CO_2 as well as measure airflow.[12] CPET provides a continuous oxygen consumption (Vo_2), including the peak Vo_2, after the anaerobic threshold has been met.[13] In addition to peak V_{O_2}, ventilatory insufficiency is measured by the expired ventilation (VE) divided by carbon dioxide production (VCO_2). This measurement is referred to as the VE/VCO_2 ratio or slope and is also used to predict outcomes in HF. A higher slope indicates a greater risk for adverse events, and may be even more powerful of a marker of HF severity than peak V_{O_2}.[14,15]

Cardiopulmonary Exercise Testing in Hypertrophic Cardiomyopathy

Exercise capacity in patients with HCM may be affected by diastolic dysfunction, restrictive physiology, LV outflow tract (LVOT) obstruction, concomitant mitral regurgitation, and sometimes reduced LV systolic function. Historically, exercise testing was considered dangerous because of the risk for arrhythmia or worsened LVOT obstruction in some patients. Several studies have shown physiologic testing, as is done during CPET, is safe. One group performed CPET and transthoracic echocardiography on 197 patients with HCM and 40 healthy controls. There were no complications during exercise, even including patients with LVOT obstruction at rest or with exercise.[16] A study of 499 consecutive patients with HCM and a resting LVOT gradient of greater than 30 mm Hg (152 patients), labile LVOT gradient (178 patients), or no gradient (178 patients) underwent a total of 959 treadmill exercise tests. There were no deaths and only 3 serious ventricular arrhythmias (0.3% of tests). Patients with obstructive HCM had a greater amount of abnormal blood pressure responses.[17] A retrospective study of adverse outcomes during CPET in 396 patients with HCM showed a 1.3% rate of ST segment changes, 0.3% (1 patient) had nonsustained ventricular tachycardia, 6.6% (26 patients) had a hypertensive response, and 5.6% (22 patients) had hypotension. There were no serious adverse outcomes of sudden death, syncope, or life-threatening arrhythmias.[18] Based on these studies as well as the growing experience of the safety of CPET in HCM, guidelines no longer advise against vigorous exercise testing in monitored settings.

CPET is used to objectively assess functional capacity and response to medications and procedural interventions for LVOT obstruction. Change in New York Heart Association functional class is often used in clinical research as an outcome, but CPET may provide a more objective assessment of functional class in patients with HCM undergoing treatment, especially in a research setting. One study of 24 patients with HCM compared the physician attributed the New York Heart Association functional class with the Kansas City Cardiomyopathy Questionnaire and the peak V_{O_2} on CPET. There was a negative correlation between the New York Heart Association functional class and the Kansas City Cardiomyopathy Questionnaire, and a statistically significant positive correlation between the Kansas City Cardiomyopathy Questionnaire and the peak V_{O_2}.[19] Given its safety and reproducibility, CPET and the derived variables such as peak V_{O_2} and VE/VCO_2 slope are being used in the assessment of response to medical and procedural interventions in HCM, and are often included as clinical endpoints in modern clinical trial design.

Cardiopulmonary Testing for Risk Stratification in Hypertrophic Cardiomyopathy

The overall prognosis of nonobstructive HCM is comparable with all-cause mortality in an age- and sex-matched population. A prospective study of 573 consecutive patients with HCM at 3 centers found that in the nonobstructive patients, mortality was just 0.5% per year with a 5-year survival rate of 99%. Of the 249 patients without LVOT obstruction, only 10% (n = 24) or 1.6% per year progressed from functional class I/II to III/IV and were subsequently referred for heart transplantation. The rates of HF progression to functional class III/IV were much higher for patients with HCM with resting obstruction (38% or 7.4% per year) and provokable obstruction (20% or 3.2% per year).[20]

Among the different phenotypes of HCM, there remains a concern for the risk of hospitalization for HF, sudden cardiac death (SCD), and low cardiac output HF. Risk assessment of SCD has historically relied on 5 clinical features: a left ventricular wall thickness of greater than 30 mm, a family history of SCD, syncope, nonsustained ventricular tachycardia, and an abnormal blood pressure response with exercise.[21,22] A more recent risk model was introduced by the HCM Outcomes Investigators, called the "HCM Risk-SCD."[23] This model was subsequently validated in a consecutive cohort of 706 patients with HCM and no prior SCD event.[24] These risk models are often focused on the decision to proceed with implantable cardioverter-defibrillators to prevent SCD.[25] In general, most HCM prognostic models do not provide insight to the risk of HF progression and need for orthotopic heart transplantation.

Although the current risk models do not take into account data from CPET, there has been an emerging body of literature on the usefulness of this test to supplement risk assessment in HCM for SCD, HF-related death, and the need for orthotopic heart transplantation. The value of CPET in the prediction of SCD was studied in a multicenter Italian study of 683 patients. During a median follow-up of 3.7 years, 25 patients had an arrhythmic event (3 SCD, 4 aborted SCD, 18 implantable cardioverter-defibrillator shocks). The VE/VCO$_2$ slope was independently associated with the study endpoint, and a cutoff value of 31 providing the optimal receiver operating curve for predicting SCD (sensitivity, 64%; specificity, 72%).[26]

Other studies suggest that CPET may not be as useful in predicting SCD as it is in predicting HF-related outcomes. In a large, single-center experience with CPET and HCM, 1898 patients between 1998 and 2010 who had undergone CPET were studied in a retrospective observational cohort for the primary outcome of death or heart transplantation. Of these, 178 patients (9.4%) had the primary outcome, with a yearly event rate of 1.6% per year. After adjusting for age, sex, left atrial size, nonsustained ventricular tachycardia, and ejection fraction, the lowest quartile of peak Vo$_2$ (<15.3 mL/kg/min) had a death/transplant event rate of 14% at 6 years and 31% at 10 years. Peak Vo$_2$ (hazard ratio, 0.81; 95% confidence interval, 0.77–0.86; P<.01) and VE/VCO$_2$ slope (hazard ratio, 1.10; 95% confidence interval, 1.08–1.13; P<.01) were significant predictors of death from HF or need for orthotopic heart transplantation, but not for SCD or implantable cardioverter-defibrillator shocks.[27] In another study of 156 patients with HCM, 21 patients (13%) achieved the composite outcome of cardiac death, orthotopic heart transplantation, and functional deterioration leading to septal reduction therapy. In an exploratory analysis of both transthoracic echocardiography and CPET variables at the time of enrollment, 3 values were independently associated with the composite outcome (mean follow-up of 27 ± 11 months): peak Vo$_2$ less than 80% predicted (hazard ratio, 4.11; P<.008), a VE/VCO$_2$ slope of greater than 34 (hazard ratio, 3.14; P<.014), and a left atrial volume index of greater than 40 mL/m^2 (hazard ratio, 3.32; P<.036).[28] CPET may also provide prognostic data on minimally symptomatic patients with HCM. In a retrospective study of 182 patients with obstructive HCM (LVOT gradient >30 mm Hg) and minimal symptoms (functional class I–II), CPET was performed and patients were followed for a mean of 4 years (±3 years). In patients with a percent predicted peak Vo$_2$ of less than 60%, the 4-year survival rate free of death or functional class III to IV symptoms was only 59%.[29]

In contrast with the HCM Risk-SCD model, which aims at predicting the risk of SCD, other groups have published risk models for prediction of HF-related events, such as progression to functional class III to IV disease, hospitalization for HF, need for septal reduction, death from HF, and orthotopic heart transplantation. One Italian multicenter study of 620 patients with HCM followed from 2007 to 2015 analyzed CPET and transthoracic echocardiography variables to create a *HYP*ertrophic *E*xercise-derived *R*isk *HF* (HYPERHF) model to predict these HF-related outcomes. In this prospective study, peak Vo$_2$, VE/VCO$_2$ slope, and left atrial diameter were independently associated with HF outcomes, which occurred in 84 patients over a median follow-up of 3.8 years. The HYPERHF equation, using these 3 variables, 2 of which require CPET, provides an estimated 5-year event rate with the best cutoff score of greater than 15% yielding a sensitivity of 86%, specificity of 72%, positive predictive value of 0.32, and negative predictive value of 0.97.[30]

Cardiopulmonary Exercise Testing and Cardiac Transplantation

As demonstrated, CPET has an emerging role in the identification of patients with HCM at risk for SCD and HF-related outcomes, such as death from low cardiac output, progression to functional class III or IV disease, hospitalization, and need for orthotopic heart transplantation. In general, the peak Vo$_2$ is very commonly used to assess prognosis of HF with a reduced ejection fraction. In a study of 114 candidates for orthotopic heart transplantation patients with advanced HF with a reduced ejection fraction, Mancini and colleagues[31] followed survival as stratified by peak Vo$_2$ achieved on CPET. Patients with a peak Vo$_2$ of less than 14 mL O$_2$ kg^{-1}min^{-1} had a very poor survival of 47% at 1 year, versus patients achieving a peak Vo$_2$ of greater than 14 mL O$_2$ kg^{-1}min^{-1}, who had a 94% survival at 1 year, an outcome similar to patients undergoing orthotopic heart transplantation. Because this study was done before the routine use of beta-blockers, a lower cutoff of 12 mL O$_2$ kg^{-1}min^{-1} is used to identity higher risk patients who may benefit from evaluation for advanced therapies, such as orthotopic heart transplantation and mechanical circulatory support.[32] Limitations of using peak Vo$_2$ for prognosis in HF include the effect of beta-blockers lowering peak Vo$_2$ and other conditions other than HF limiting exercise, such as peripheral arterial disease, arthritis, and poor motivation. As mentioned, the higher the measured VE/VCO$_2$, the worse the outcomes are in HF. In the 2016 International Society for Heart Lung Transplantation listing criteria, a VE/VCO$_2$ slope of greater than 35 was added as a listing criterion for orthotopic heart transplantation.[32]

The use of CPET for prognosis in HF with preserved ejection fraction, including patients with HCM with normal ejection fraction, has been less studied. There are several indications that CPET variables are similar in HF with preserved ejection fraction and HF with a reduced ejection fraction, and that a reduced peak Vo$_2$ can still identify patients with HF with preserved ejection fraction who are at higher risk for death and readmission.[33–35] Advanced HF symptoms resulting from a small stroke volume and low cardiac output, despite the presence of a normal ejection fraction, are common in HCM. CPET is useful in identifying these very symptomatic patients by demonstrating their physiologic limitation to exercise and validating referral for orthotopic heart transplantation.

Guideline Recommendations for the Use of Cardiopulmonary Testing in Hypertrophic Cardiomyopathy

The 2011 American College of Cardiology/American Heart Association HCM guidelines recommend treadmill exercise testing to determine functional capacity and assess the response to medications and other interventions in HCM such as alcohol septal ablation and surgical myectomy for LVOT obstruction (Class IIa recommendation). Combining exercise testing with echocardiography is useful to identify a provokable LVOT gradient or worsening mitral regurgitation. In regards to metabolic stress testing (CPET), guidelines suggest that the role is uncertain, but it may be helpful in quantifying functional capacity, especially if the clinical history is unreliable.[22] The more recent 2014 European Society of Cardiology guidelines recommend CPET for all patients being considered for orthotopic heart transplantation or mechanical support (Class Ib), for patients with HCM regardless of symptoms to assess severity of disease (Class IIa), and in patients being evaluated for interventions for LVOT obstruction (Class IIa).[21]

SUMMARY

HCM, which has a wide variability in its phenotype and clinical course, may require advanced testing including cardiac catheterization, endomyocardial biopsy, and CPET. Right and left heart catheterization provides essential hemodynamic data to guide treatment of patients with HCM, identifies patients who might benefit from septal reduction therapy, and assesses for other comorbidities such as coronary artery disease or pulmonary hypertension that may be contributing to symptoms. Pathologic analysis of HCM reveals ventricular hypertrophy, myocardial disarray, and endocardial and interstitial fibrosis. Routine endomyocardial biopsy is not recommended in the evaluation of a patient with suspected HCM, unless other conditions that cause ventricular hypertrophy need to be ruled out, such as metabolic storage diseases or amyloid. CPET, which relies on vigorous treadmill or bicycle exercise that was once considered a relative contraindication in HCM, has now been shown to be safe and efficacious in the assessment of risk in these patients. It may also provide more objective endpoints in clinical research studies. Specifically, a low peak Vo$_2$ (<12 mL O$_2$ kg^{-1}min^{-1} if on a beta-blocker) and a high VE/VCO$_2$ slope of greater than 35 identify patients at risk for death, progression of HF, and need for consideration of cardiac transplantation. Future clinical trial design is likely to include CPET variables as a clinical outcome. Familiarity and further research into the nuances of cardiac catheterization and CPET may help to guide therapy for patients with HCM and advance our understanding of the multiple phenotypes and physiologies of this condition.

REFERENCES

1. Semsarian C, Ingles J, Maron MS, et al. New perspectives on the prevalence of hypertrophic cardiomyopathy. J Am Coll Cardiol 2015;65(12): 1249–54.
2. Sorajja P, Borlaug BA, Dimas VV, et al. SCAI/HFSA clinical expert consensus document on the use of invasive hemodynamics for the diagnosis and management of cardiovascular disease. Catheter Cardiovasc Interv 2017;89(7):E233–47.
3. Khouzam RN, Naidu SS. Current status and future perspectives on alcohol septal ablation for hypertrophic obstructive cardiomyopathy. Curr Cardiol Rep 2014;16(5):478.
4. Shenouda J, Silber D, Subramaniam M, et al. Evaluation and management of concomitant hypertrophic obstructive cardiomyopathy and valvular aortic stenosis. Curr Treat Options Cardiovasc Med 2016; 18(3):17.
5. Teare D. Asymmetrical hypertrophy of the heart in young adults. Brit Heart J 1958;20:1–8.
6. Marian AJ, Braunwald E. Hypertrophic cardiomyopathy: genetics, pathogenesis, clinical manifestations, diagnosis, and therapy. Circ Res 2017; 121(7):749–70.
7. Kamisago M, Sharma SD, DePalma SR, et al. Mutations in sarcomere protein genes as a cause of

dilated cardiomyopathy. N Engl J Med 2000; 343(23):1688–96.

8. Teo EP, Teoh JG, Hung J. Mitral valve and papillary muscle abnormalities in hypertrophic obstructive cardiomyopathy. Curr Opin Cardiol 2015;30(5): 475–82.

9. Abecasis J, Gouveia R, Castro M, et al. Surgical pathology of subaortic septal myectomy: histology skips over clinical diagnosis. Cardiovasc Pathol 2018;33:32–8.

10. Weiner DA, Ryan TJ, McCabe CH, et al. Prognostic importance of a clinical profile and exercise test in medically treated patients with coronary artery disease. J Am Coll Cardiol 1984;3(3):772–9.

11. Huelsmann M, Stefenelli T, Berger R, et al. Prognostic impact of workload in patients with congestive heart failure. Am Heart J 2002;143(2):308–12.

12. Neuberg GW, Friedman SH, Weiss MB, et al. Cardiopulmonary exercise testing. The clinical value of gas exchange data. Arch Intern Med 1988;148(10): 2221–6.

13. Malhotra R, Bakken K, D'Elia E. Cardiopulmonary exercise testing in heart failure. Curr Probl Cardiol 2015;40(8):322–72. Available at: http://www. embase.com/search/results?subaction=viewrecord& from=export&id=L605263703%5Cnhttps://doi.org/10. 1016/j.cpcardiol.2015.01.009%5Cnhttp://sfx.library. uu.nl/utrecht?sid=EMBASE&issn=15356280&id= doi:10.1016%2Fj.cpcardiol.2015.01.009&atitle= Cardiopul.

14. Guazzi M, Adams V, Conraads V, et al. Clinical recommendations for cardiopulmonary exercise testing data assessment in specific patient populations. Eur Heart J 2012;33(23):2917–27.

15. Arena R, Myers J, Abella J, et al. Development of a ventilatory classification system in patients with heart failure. Circulation 2007;115(18):2410–7.

16. Re F, Zachara E, Avella A, et al. Dissecting functional impairment in hypertrophic cardiomyopathy by dynamic assessment of diastolic reserve and outflow obstruction: a combined cardiopulmonary-echocardiographic study. Int J Cardiol 2017;227: 743–50.

17. Sorensen LL, Liang HY, Pinheiro A, et al. Safety profile and utility of treadmill exercise in patients with high-gradient hypertrophic cardiomyopathy. Am Heart J 2017;184:47–54.

18. Blank C, Pfeiffer B, Neugebauer A, et al. Safety of cardiopulmonary exercise test in hypertrophic cardiomyopathy. Eur Heart J 2009;Conference:81. Available at: http://ovidsp.ovid.com/ ovidweb.cgi?T=JS&CSC=Y&NEWS=N&PAGE= fulltext&D=emed9&AN=70353419http://oxfordsfx. hosted.exlibrisgroup.com/oxford?sid=OVID:embase& id=pmid:&id=doi:10.1093/eurheartj/ehp413&issn= 0195-668X&isbn=&volume=30&issue=1&spage= 81&pages=81&date=2.

19. Huff CM, Turer AT, Wang A. Correlations between physician-perceived functional status, patient-perceived health status, and cardiopulmonary exercise results in hypertrophic cardiomyopathy. Qual Life Res 2013;22(3):647–52.

20. Maron MS, Rowin EJ, Olivotto I, et al. Contemporary natural history and management of nonobstructive hypertrophic cardiomyopathy. J Am Coll Cardiol 2016;67(12):1399–409.

21. Authors/Task Force members AF, Elliott PM, Anastasakis A, et al. 2014 ESC guidelines on diagnosis and management of hypertrophic cardiomyopathy: the task force for the diagnosis and management of hypertrophic cardiomyopathy of the European Society of Cardiology (ESC). Eur Heart J 2014;35(39):2733–79.

22. Gersh BJ, Maron BJ, Bonow RO, et al. 2011 ACCF/ AHA guideline for the diagnosis and treatment of hypertrophic cardiomyopathy. Circulation 2011; 124(24):e783–831. Available at: http://circ.ahajournals. org/content/124/24/e783.abstract.

23. O'Mahony C, Jichi F, Pavlou M, et al. A novel clinical risk prediction model for sudden cardiac death in hypertrophic cardiomyopathy (HCM Risk-SCD). Eur Heart J 2014;35(30):2010–20.

24. Vriesendorp PA, Schinkel AFL, Liebregts M, et al. Validation of the 2014 European Society of Cardiology Guidelines risk prediction model for the primary prevention of sudden cardiac death in hypertrophic cardiomyopathy. Circ Arrhythm Electrophysiol 2015; 8(4):829–35.

25. Maron BJ. Risk stratification and role of implantable defibrillators for prevention of sudden death in patients with hypertrophic cardiomyopathy. Circ J 2010;74(11):2271–82. Available at: http://www. embase.com/search/results?subaction=viewrecord& from=export&id=L359972622%5Cnhttp://www.jstage. jst.go.jp/article/circj/74/11/2271/_pdf%5Cnhttps://doi. org/10.1253/circj.CJ-10-0921%5Cnhttp://sfx.library. uu.nl/utrecht?sid=EMBASE&issn=13469843&id=.

26. Magri D, Limongelli G, Re F, et al. Cardiopulmonary exercise test and sudden cardiac death risk in hypertrophic cardiomyopathy. Heart 2016;102(8): 602–9.

27. Coats CJ, Rantell K, Bartnik A, et al. Cardiopulmonary exercise testing and prognosis in hypertrophic cardiomyopathy. Circ Hear Fail 2015;8(6): 1022–31.

28. Finocchiaro G, Haddad F, Knowles JW, et al. Cardiopulmonary responses and prognosis in hypertrophic cardiomyopathy. JACC Hear Fail 2015; 3(5):408–18.

29. Sorajja P, Allison T, Hayes C, et al. Prognostic utility of metabolic exercise testing in minimally symptomatic patients with obstructive hypertrophic cardiomyopathy. Am J Cardiol 2012;109(10): 1494–8.

30. Magrì D, Re F, Limongelli G, et al. Heart failure progression in hypertrophic cardiomyopathy– possible insights from cardiopulmonary exercise testing. Circ J 2016;80(10):2204–11.

31. Mancini DM, Eisen H, Kussmaul W, et al. Value of peak exercise oxygen consumption for optimal timing of cardiac transplantation in ambulatory patients with heart failure. Circulation 1991;83(3): 778–86.

32. Mehra MR, Canter CE, Hannan MM, et al. The 2016 International Society for Heart Lung Transplantation listing criteria for heart transplantation: a 10-year update. J Hear Lung Transplant 2016;35(1): 1–23.

33. Palau P, Domínguez E, Núñez E, et al. Peak exercise oxygen uptake predicts recurrent admissions in heart failure with preserved ejection fraction. Rev Esp Cardiol (Engl Ed) 2018;71(4): 250–6.

34. Guazzi M. Cardiopulmonary exercise testing in heart failure preserved ejection fraction: time to expand the paradigm in the prognostic algorithm. Am Heart J 2016;174:164–6.

35. Guazzi M, Labate V, Cahalin LP, et al. Cardiopulmonary exercise testing reflects similar pathophysiology and disease severity in heart failure patients with reduced and preserved ejection fraction. Eur J Prev Cardiol 2014;21(7):847–54.

Choice of Septal Reduction Therapies and Alcohol Septal Ablation

Michael A. Fifer, MD

KEYWORDS

- Alcohol septal ablation • Hypertrophic cardiomyopathy • Hypertrophic obstructive cardiomyopathy
- Septal ablation • Septal reduction therapy

KEY POINTS

- Septal reduction therapy is appropriate for patients with hypertrophic obstructive cardiomyopathy (HOCM) who have symptoms that are refractory to optimal medical therapy, and that interfere importantly enough with lifestyle that patients are willing to assume the risks of invasive procedures.
- Given the overall comparable outcomes after septal ablation and septal myectomy, for many patients, there is equipoise between the two procedures.
- Septal ablation is performed with standard angioplasty guiding catheters, guidewires, and balloon catheters.
- Because atrioventricular block constitutes the major morbidity of the procedure, temporary pacemaker placement is required in patients without permanent devices.
- In the Euro-ASA registry, NYHA functional class fell from 2.9 ± 0.5 to 1.6 ± 0.7 and gradient from 67 ± 36 to 16 ± 21 mm Hg at mean 3.9-year follow-up after septal ablation.

PATIENT SELECTION FOR SEPTAL REDUCTION THERAPY

In most symptomatic patients with hypertrophic obstructive cardiomyopathy (HOCM), symptoms are adequately controlled with negative inotropic medications (ß-blockers, calcium channel blockers, and disopyramide) alone or in combination.[1,2] In patients with HOCM and symptoms refractory to optimal medical therapy, septal reduction therapy (SRT) with either alcohol septal ablation or surgical septal myectomy may be considered.

The 2011 American College of Cardiology Foundation (ACCF)/American Heart Association (AHA) guidelines[3] specify that SRT should be performed:

- By experienced operators, that is, those with cumulative case volumes of at least 20 procedures or working in a dedicated

hypertrophic cardiomyopathy (HCM) program with a cumulative total of at least 50 procedures.
- In patients with severe (usually New York Heart Association [NYHA] functional class III or IV) dyspnea or chest pain, or exertional syncope or presyncope that interferes with everyday activity despite optimal medical therapy.
- In the presence of a left ventricular outflow tract (LVOT) gradient of greater than or equal to 50 mm Hg at rest or with physiologic provocation
- In the presence of septal thickness "sufficient to perform the procedure safely and effectively," generally greater than or equal to 15 mm, per these and the 2014 European Society of Cardiology (ESC) guidelines.[4]

Disclosure Statement: Dr M.A. Fifer serves on the Scientific Advisory Board of MyoKardia, Inc.
Hypertrophic Cardiomyopathy Program, Massachusetts General Hospital, Harvard Medical School, 55 Fruit Street, GRB 800, Boston, MA 02114, USA
E-mail address: fifer.michael@mgh.harvard.edu

Cardiol Clin 37 (2019) 83–93
https://doi.org/10.1016/j.ccl.2018.08.009
0733-8651/19/© 2018 Elsevier Inc. All rights reserved.

Effect of Procedure Volume on Outcomes

Using a national inpatient database, Kim and colleagues[5] reported in 2016 that many US hospitals performed far fewer SRT procedures than those recommended by the ACCF/AHA guidelines, and that mortality and other complication rates were inversely related to procedure volume, in particular for septal myectomy. Reporting for the Euro-ASA Registry, Veselka and coworkers[6] showed that, within each institution, outcomes in the first 50 procedures were inferior to those in subsequent procedures. These data support the consolidation of SRT procedures in high-volume centers associated with multidisciplinary HCM programs.[7]

What About Patients in New York Heart Association Functional Class II?

Because patients in NYHA functional class II have, by definition, symptoms during "ordinary physical activity,"[8] some of these are also appropriate candidates for SRT. Patients in functional class II are, in fact, often managed with either septal ablation[9–11] or septal myectomy.[9,10,12] Veselka and colleagues[13] reported the outcomes in 161 NYHA functional class II patients (11% of the total population undergoing septal ablation) in the Euro-ASA registry. All of these patients "had significantly reduced quality of life attributed to dyspnea." At latest follow-up, 69% of the patients were in NYHA functional class I. These findings support consideration of SRT in patients in NYHA functional class II.[14]

What About Patients in New York Heart Association Functional Class I?

Sorajja and colleagues[15] have reported that the presence of a substantial LVOT gradient is associated with an adverse prognosis even in patients with no or mild symptoms and that patients who have undergone SRT have a favorable prognosis.[16] Although these authors did not conclude that patients with no or minimal symptoms should therefore undergo SRT, others have raised this possibility.[13] In the absence of conclusive data to indicate that reducing or abolishing the gradient improves prognosis, however, SRT should not be offered to adult patients, even those with large gradients, if they have no or mild symptoms.

Septal Reduction Therapy for Overt Congestive Heart Failure

HOCM patients with overt congestive heart failure are perhaps at the other end of the symptom spectrum. Although the exertional dyspnea that characterizes symptomatic patients with HOCM is often termed a "heart failure" symptom, it is generally distinct from the congestive symptoms that typically characterize patients with other causes of heart failure. A minority of patients with HCM, including some with HOCM, however, do have the symptoms and signs of congestive heart failure. Mechanisms responsible for pulmonary congestion in HOCM include abnormal diastolic left ventricular (LV) function associated with hypertrophy and, in some patients, fibrosis; and mitral regurgitation associated with systolic anterior motion of the mitral valve.[17]

As pointed out by McKay and Nagueh,[18] SRT may lower left atrial pressure via regression of LV hypertrophy and amelioration of mitral regurgitation. Kitamura and colleagues,[19] however, reported that diuretic usage before septal ablation was a predictor of the need for repeat ablation.

Thus, SRT is appropriate for patients with HOCM who have symptoms (exertional dyspnea, angina, and/or "hemodynamic" syncope) that are refractory to optimal medical therapy and that interfere importantly enough with lifestyle (independently of NYHA functional class) that patients are willing to assume the morbidity and mortality of invasive procedures.

Means of Gradient Provocation

SRT is appropriate for patients with either resting or provoked LVOT obstruction[20,21]; in fact, the three patients in Sigwart's initial series had provoked rather than resting obstruction.[22] In patients without resting LVOT gradients of at least 50 mm Hg, provocative maneuvers may bring out a gradient. In the echocardiography laboratory, LVOT gradients may be provoked by the Valsalva maneuver, exercise, or amyl nitrite.[23] In the cardiac catheterization laboratory, gradients may be provoked by the Valsalva maneuver, postextrasystolic potentiation, or nitroglycerin.[24] Whereas the ACCF/AHA guidelines recommend "physiologic" provocation, it may be appropriate in selected cases to use isoproterenol or nitroglycerin in the cardiac catheterization laboratory for gradient provocation.[25]

Wall Thickness

The ACCF/AHA guidelines state that a requirement for SRT is the presence of "targeted anterior septal thickness sufficient to perform the procedure safely and effectively in the judgment of the individual operator," and, more specifically, that, "because of the potential for creating a ventricular septal defect, septal ablation should not be performed if the target septal thickness is ≤15 mm."[3] The 2014 ESC guidelines state that "in general, the risk of ventriculoseptal defect following septal alcohol ablation and septal myectomy is higher in patients with mild hypertrophy (≤16 mm) at the point of the mitral leaflet–septal contact."[4]

Although the creation of a ventricular septal defect complicates 1% to 2% of septal myectomy procedures[26] and, more rarely, septal ablation,[27] there are no systematic data relating the risk to preprocedural septal thickness. In some patients with modest degrees of septal hypertrophy, surgical mitral valve replacement or repair is sometimes performed as an alternative to SRT, whether or not intrinsic abnormalities of the mitral valve are identified,[28] although this practice has been challenged.[29] Recently, transcatheter clipping of the mitral valve has been proposed for management of these patients.[30]

CHOICE OF SEPTAL REDUCTION THERAPIES
Concomitant Cardiac Conditions

In some cases, HOCM is associated with intrinsic abnormalities of the mitral valve. These and other patients who require concomitant valve surgery or coronary bypass grafting should undergo septal myectomy rather than septal ablation. Surgery should also be considered for patients with atrial fibrillation who might benefit from a concomitant maze procedure.

Concomitant Noncardiac Conditions

Comorbidities, such as lung and liver disease, generally increase the risk of cardiac surgery more than the risk of interventional catheterization laboratory procedures, and thus favor septal ablation over septal myectomy.

Age

The benefit of alcohol septal ablation in older patients is similar to that in younger patients.[11,31] Because the risks of cardiac surgery generally increase with age, ablation may offer an advantage in older patients. With regard to younger patients, the ACCF/AHA guidelines state that "alcohol septal ablation...is discouraged in adults less than 40 years of age if myectomy is a viable option."[3] A recent report, however, indicates that septal ablation is effective and safe in younger patients,[32] suggesting that the guidelines should be updated in this regard.[33]

Wall Thickness

The ACCF/AHA guidelines state that "the effectiveness of alcohol septal ablation is uncertain in patients with HCM with marked (ie, >30 mm) septal hypertrophy, and therefore the procedure is generally discouraged in such patients."[3] The 2014 ESC guidelines state that "septal ablation may be less effective in...patients with very severe hypertrophy (≥30 mm), but systematic data are lacking."[4]

Data with regard to the success of septal ablation in patients with marked septal hypertrophy are mixed. Lu and colleagues[34] performed echocardiography and cardiac MRI before and echocardiography 6 months after septal ablation in 102 patients, which was deemed successful in 73 patients. Mean preablation echocardiographic septal thickness was 23 in the success and 28 in the failure groups ($P<.001$). Combined preablation basal anterior and basal anteroseptal wall thickness as assessed by MRI was 47 mm in the success and 55 in the failure groups ($P<.001$). Yang and colleagues,[35] however, found that the success of septal ablation was not adversely affected by the presence of echocardiographic septal thickness greater than or equal to 30 mm. Kitamura and coworkers[19] found that the success of septal ablation was predicted less by the extent of anteroseptal hypertrophy than by an extended hypertrophy score reflecting the extent of hypertrophy in basal segments apart from the anteroseptal segments.

Conduction System Disease and Pacemakers

By an unfortunate coincidence, the blood supply to the upper septum is shared by the intraventricular conduction system (**Fig. 1**). The incidence of

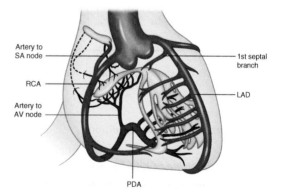

Fig. 1. Schematic diagram of blood supply to cardiac conduction system. The first septal branch of the left anterior descending (LAD) coronary artery supplies a critical portion of the interventricular conduction system. AV, atrioventricular; PDA, posterior descending artery; RCA, right coronary artery; SA, sinoatrial. (*Adapted from* Harthorne JW, Pohost GM. Electrical therapy of cardiac dysrhythmias. In: Levine HJ, editor. Clinical cardiovascular physiology. New York: Grune and Stratton; 1976. p. 854; with permission.)

right bundle branch block after alcohol septal ablation is approximately 50%,[36] so that patients with preexisting left bundle branch block are at particular risk of complete heart block after septal ablation. Conversely, the incidence of left bundle branch block after septal myectomy is approximately 50%[37]; thus, patients with preexisting right bundle branch block are at particular risk of complete heart block after septal myectomy.

The principal morbidity and a component of the mortality of septal ablation is complete heart block. Patients with pacemakers (or implanted cardioverter defibrillators) are thus at lower risk of complications of the procedure.

How to Choose

Based on these considerations, factors favoring one SRT over the other are summarized in **Box 1**. For patients without these factors, the choice of SRT is more challenging. There have been no prospective randomized trials comparing septal ablation with septal myectomy. Non-randomized comparisons are summarized in **Table 1** and meta-analyses are shown in **Table 2**.

Given the overall comparable outcomes after septal ablation and septal myectomy, there is, for many if not most patients, equipoise between the two procedures. Indeed, although the 2011 ACCF/AHA guidelines state that myectomy is the "first consideration" for most patients,[3] the ESC guidelines, published 3 years later, are more even-handed.[4] Septal ablation has the potential for greater patient satisfaction because of the absence of a surgical incision and need for general anesthesia, the lower amount of pain, and the much shorter recovery time. Cardiologists and their

patients are confronted by the choice between percutaneous transcatheter and surgical therapies much more often in coronary artery disease than in HOCM. In the setting of coronary artery disease, most patients for whom either procedure would be appropriate choose percutaneous coronary intervention over coronary artery bypass grafting. Similarly, most "gray area" patients with HOCM choose septal ablation over septal myectomy.[38] Patients are of course influenced by the information presented to them by physicians and the manner in which it is presented.

THE SEPTAL ABLATION PROCEDURE
Initial Septal Ablation Procedures

Transcatheter ablation of the septum with ethanol was introduced by Sigwart in 1994 at Royal Brompton Hospital.[22] The first patient had labile LVOT obstruction and severe symptoms despite ß-blockade. Peak creatine kinase was 2500 U/L. She was discharged 3 days after septal ablation, and was asymptomatic 10 months later.

Indications

Indications for septal ablation are summarized in **Box 2**.

Technique

Because atrioventricular block constitutes the major morbidity of septal ablation, temporary pacemaker placement is required in patients without permanent devices. In patients with lower or absent resting gradients, higher gradients may be provoked with the Valsalva maneuver, postextrasystolic potentiation, nitroglycerin,[24] dobutamine, or isoproterenol.[25]

Septal ablation is performed with standard angioplasty guiding catheters, guidewires, and balloon catheters. The target territory is the basal septum at the point of systolic contact by the anterior leaflet of the mitral valve. This segment is usually but not always supplied by the first septal branch of the left anterior descending coronary artery. Proper vessel selection is determined by myocardial contrast echocardiography (**Fig. 2**).[47–49] Myocardial contrast may be achieved with agitated radiographic contrast or an echocardiographic contrast agent. The routine use of myocardial contrast echocardiography in septal ablation has resulted in decreases in ethanol volume and complication rates.

Once the target vessel is selected, pure ethanol is slowly infused via the balloon catheter (with the balloon inflated). The acute efficacy of ethanol infusion is judged by reduction of the LVOT

> **Box 1**
> **Factors favoring septal ablation or septal myectomy**
>
> *Ablation*
> - Comorbid noncardiac conditions
> - Older
> - Preexisting right bundle branch block
> - Prior pacemaker (or implantable cardioverter defibrillator)
>
> *Myectomy*
> - Other "surgical" cardiac conditions, such as intrinsic mitral valve abnormalities
> - Younger
> - Thicker
> - Preexisting left bundle branch block

Table 1
Studies comparing efficacy and safely of septal ablation and septal myectomy

Authors	Institution	Number of Patients	How Triaged	Efficacy	Safety
Nagueh et al,[9] 2001	Baylor (ablation), Mayo Clinic (myectomy)	41 ablation, 41 myectomy	Institutional preference	No difference in NYHA functional class, exercise capacity, or gradient	Mortality 2% ablation vs 0% myectomy; PM 22% ablation vs 2% myectomy
Qin et al,[39] 2001	Cleveland Clinic	25 ablation, 26 myectomy	Age, comorbid conditions, need for concomitant surgery	No difference in NYHA functional class; >50% gradient reduction in 76% ablation vs 100% myectomy	No mortality; PM in 24% ablation vs 8% myectomy
Firoozi et al,[10] 2002	St. George's Hospital	20 ablation, 24 myectomy	Age, patient and physician choice	No difference in NYHA functional class or gradient; exercise capacity better after myectomy	Mortality 5% ablation vs 4% myectomy; PM 15% ablation vs 4% myectomy
Ralph-Edwards et al,[12] 2005	Toronto General Hospital	54 ablation, 48 myectomy	Age, patient and physician choice	NYHA functional class I or II in 41% ablation vs 72% myectomy	Late mortality in 11% ablation vs 0% myectomy
Sorajja et al,[40] 2008	Mayo Clinic	123 ablation, 123 myectomy	Comorbid conditions, patient choice	No difference in survival free of severe symptoms	No difference in mortality; PM 23% ablation vs 2% myectomy
ten Cate et al,[41] 2010	Thoraxcenter	91 ablation, 40 myectomy	Comorbid conditions, need for concomitant surgery, patient choice	Not reported	Higher rate of cardiac death or aborted sudden death after ablation
Steggerda et al,[42] 2014	The Netherlands	161 ablation, 102 myectomy	Need for concomitant surgery, patient choice	No difference in survival, symptoms, or heart failure hospitalizations	No difference in mortality or PM; more tamponade in myectomy group
Vriesendorp et al,[43] 2014	The Netherlands, Belgium	316 ablation, 250 myectomy	Not specified	No difference in gradient reduction, but more repeat procedures after ablation	No difference in mortality; more ICD discharges after ablation

Abbreviations: ICD, implantable cardioverter defibrillator; PM, pacemaker.
Adapted from Fifer MA. Most fully informed patients choose septal ablation over septal myectomy. Circulation 2007;116(2):211; with permission.

Table 2
Meta-analyses comparing efficacy and safely of septal ablation and septal myectomy

Authors	Studies	Efficacy	Safety
Agarwal et al,[44] 2010	12 comparative studies	No difference in NYHA functional class or gradient	No difference in mortality or ventricular arrhythmias; more PM after ablation
Leonardi et al,[45] 2010	19 ablation and 8 myectomy studies	No difference in NYHA functional class; higher gradient after ablation	No difference in unadjusted mortality, SCD; lower adjusted mortality and SCD after ablation; more PM after ablation
Liebregts et al,[46] 2015	24 studies including 11 ablation and 16 myectomy cohorts	More reintervention after ablation	No difference in mortality or SCD; more PM after ablation

Abbreviations: PM, pacemaker; SCD, sudden cardiac death.

gradient, usually to less than 20 mm Hg (**Fig. 3**) and by echocardiographic visualization that the consequently echodense segment of myocardium "covers the waterfront" of possible mitral valve contact. In most cases, the total volume infused is 1 to 2 mL; studies have indicated that these lower volumes are effective and that the complication rates associated with them are lower than with higher volumes.[50,51]

Peak creatine kinase is approximately 500 U/L per milliliter ethanol injected. In patients with failed septal ablation who subsequently undergo septal myectomy, we have found pathologic evidence of necrosis of the vascular endothelium (**Fig. 4**),

suggesting that ethanol is toxic to the coronary circulation and the myocardium.[52]

Results

In a sizable subset of patients, the LVOT gradient response is triphasic, with immediate reduction, early reappearance, and, by 3 months after the procedure, sustained fall.[53,54] This sequence suggests that myocardial stunning may be responsible in large part for the immediate reduction in gradient. After recovery from stunning, ultimate gradient reduction is associated with remodeling of the septum with an increase in LVOT area.[55] Improvement in symptoms occurs over the same 3-month period. In the Euro-ASA registry, NYHA functional class fell from 2.9 ± 0.5 to 1.6 ± 0.7 and LVOT gradient from 67 ± 36 to 16 ± 21 mm Hg at mean 3.9-year follow-up.[56]

With the reduction of LVOT obstruction, there are concomitant decreases in the degree of mitral regurgitation and the size of the left atrium.[47] Amelioration of the systolic pressure overload brings about regression of hypertrophy throughout the LV (**Fig. 5**).[57–59] Reduction in LVOT gradient and regression of LV hypertrophy are accompanied by an improvement in diastolic LV function,[47,60] which correlates with an increase in exercise capacity.[61] Furthermore, septal ablation brings about decreases in right ventricular mass,[58] possibly as a result of a decrease in right ventricular afterload.

Box 2
Indications for alcohol septal ablation

- Symptoms that interfere substantially with lifestyle despite optimal medical therapy
- Septal thickness ≥15 to 16 mm
- Resting left ventricular outflow tract gradient ≥30 to 50 mm Hg or provoked gradient ≥50 to 60 mm Hg
- Adequately sized and accessible septal branches supplying the target myocardial segment
- Absence of important intrinsic abnormality of mitral valve and of other conditions for which cardiac surgery is indicated
- Absolute or relative contraindication to cardiac surgery or patient preference for septal ablation when both options are reasonable and patient has been fully informed regarding benefits and risk of both procedures

From Fifer MA, Sigwart U. Controversies in cardiovascular medicine. Hypertrophic obstructive cardiomyopathy: alcohol septal ablation. Eur Heart J 2011;32(9):1064; with permission.

Complications

The incidence of temporary complete atrioventricular block during septal ablation is approximately 50%.[36,47,62,63] Following the procedure, right bundle branch block is present in approximately half of patients.[36,37,47,48,63] The rate of permanent

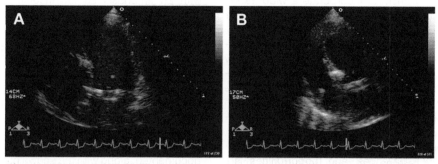

Fig. 2. Use of myocardial contrast echocardiography to select the appropriate septal branch for ethanol administration. (*A*) Contrast injected into a large septal perforator led to enhancement of the septum at the midventricular level and on the right ventricular side of the septum. Therefore, ethanol was not administered into this branch. (*B*) Contrast injected into a smaller perforator (more proximal in the left anterior descending coronary artery) indicated a more discrete target area. Alcohol septal ablation was performed via this branch. (*From* Sanborn DMY, Sigwart U, Fifer MA. Patient selection for alcohol septal ablation for hypertrophic obstructive cardiomyopathy: clinical and echocardiographic evaluation. Interv Cardiol 2012;4(3):355; with permission.)

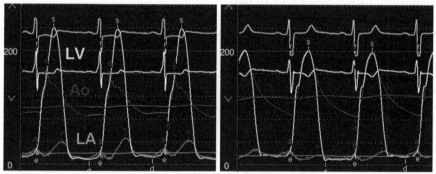

Fig. 3. Left ventricular (LV), aortic (Ao), and left atrial (LA) pressures before (*left*) and immediately after (*right*) alcohol septal ablation. (*From* Fifer MA, Sigwart U. Controversies in cardiovascular medicine. Hypertrophic obstructive cardiomyopathy: alcohol septal ablation. Eur Heart J 2011;32(9):1061; with permission.)

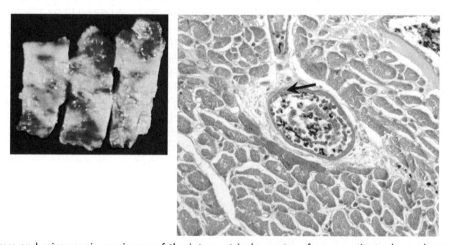

Fig. 4. Gross and microscopic specimens of the interventricular septum from a patient who underwent septal myectomy after unsuccessful alcohol septal ablation. (*Left*) The myocardium is yellow, and thus necrotic. (*Right*) Both myocytes (*yellow arrow*) and vascular endothelial cells (*black arrow*) are devoid of nuclei, indicating necrosis (hematoxylin-eosin, original magnification ×100). (*From* Baggish AL, Smith RN, Palacios I, et al. Pathologic effects of alcohol septal ablation for hypertrophic obstructive cardiomyopathy. Heart 2006;92(12):1776; with permission.)

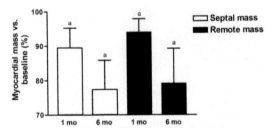

Fig. 5. Regression of LV hypertrophy after septal ablation, including in segments remote from ablation site. [a] P<.01 versus baseline. (*From* van Dockum WG, Beek AM, ten Cate FJ, et al. Early onset and progression of left ventricular remodeling after alcohol septal ablation in hypertrophic obstructive cardiomyopathy. Circulation 2005;111(19):2507; with permission.)

pacemaker placement has fallen with the use of lower dosages of ethanol, with registry data indicating a rate of 12%.[56] Much less common complications of the procedure include remote myocardial infarction caused by aberrant ethanol injection[64] or collateral circulation[65] and in-hospital sustained ventricular tachyarrhythmias.[66]

In-hospital mortality is approximately 1%.[5,27,56,67] The theoretic concern that, after septal ablation, arrhythmic sudden death caused by superimposition of a myocardial infarction on a cardiomyopathic substrate would be a common occurrence has not been realized.[68,69] The ESC sudden cardiac death risk score seems to be valid after septal ablation.[70] Following septal ablation, there may be a reduction in the sudden cardiac death risk profile.[69] Long-term mortality after the procedure is similar to that of patients who have undergone septal myectomy[16] and the general population.[16,71]

Newer Techniques

Intracardiac in place of transthoracic echocardiography has been used to guide septal ablation.[72] Septal ablation has been applied in some cases to patients with midventricular rather than LVOT obstruction.[73] Coil embolization,[74] radiofrequency ablation,[75] and cryoablation[76] have been proposed as alternatives to ethanol infusion. An intriguing alternative, particular in patients with only modest septal hypertrophy, is percutaneous placement of a mitral valve clip.[30] Alcohol septal ablation has been used for patients undergoing transcatheter aortic[77] or mitral[78] valve implantation[77] who have, or are deemed to be at risk for, LVOT obstruction following these procedures. An active-fixation pacemaker lead, placed via the transjugular approach, has been incorporated in many centers and allows for lead stability, earlier ambulation, and prolonged monitoring in some patients.

REFERENCES

1. Fifer MA, Vlahakes GJ. Management of symptoms in hypertrophic cardiomyopathy. Circulation 2008; 117(3):429–39.
2. Rothman RD, Baggish AL, O'Callaghan C, et al. Management strategy in 249 consecutive patients with obstructive hypertrophic cardiomyopathy referred to a dedicated program. Am J Cardiol 2012;110(8):1169–74.
3. Gersh BJ, Maron BJ, Bonow RO, et al. 2011 ACCF/AHA guideline for the diagnosis and treatment of hypertrophic cardiomyopathy: a report of the American College of Cardiology Foundation/American Heart Association Task Force on practice guidelines. Circulation 2011;124(24):e783–831.
4. Elliott PM, Anastasakis A, Borger MA, et al. 2014 ESC guidelines on diagnosis and management of hypertrophic cardiomyopathy: the Task Force for the diagnosis and management of hypertrophic cardiomyopathy of the European Society of Cardiology (ESC). Eur Heart J 2014;35(39):2733–79.
5. Kim LK, Swaminathan RV, Looser P, et al. Hospital volume outcomes after septal myectomy and alcohol septal ablation for treatment of obstructive hypertrophic cardiomyopathy: US nationwide inpatient database, 2003-2011. JAMA Cardiol 2016; 1(3):324–32.
6. Veselka J, Faber L, Jensen MK, et al. Effect of institutional experience on outcomes of alcohol septal ablation for hypertrophic obstructive cardiomyopathy. Can J Cardiol 2018;34(1):16–22.
7. Naidu SS. Performance volume thresholds for alcohol septal ablation in treating hypertrophic cardiomyopathy: guidelines, competency statements, and now data. Can J Cardiol 2018;34(1):13–5.
8. The Criteria Committee of the New York Heart Association. Nomenclature and criteria for diagnosis of disease of the heart and great vessels. Boston: Little Brown & Co; 1994. p. 253–6.
9. Nagueh SF, Ommen SR, Lakkis NM, et al. Comparison of ethanol septal reduction therapy with surgical myectomy for the treatment of hypertrophic obstructive cardiomyopathy. J Am Coll Cardiol 2001;38(6):1701–6.
10. Firoozi S, Elliott PM, Sharma S, et al. Septal myotomy-myectomy and transcoronary septal alcohol ablation in hypertrophic obstructive cardiomyopathy. A comparison of clinical, haemodynamic and exercise outcomes. Eur Heart J 2002;23(20): 1617–24.
11. Gietzen FH, Leuner CJ, Obergassel L, et al. Transcoronary ablation of septal hypertrophy for hypertrophic obstructive cardiomyopathy: feasibility, clinical benefit, and short term results in elderly patients. Heart 2004;90(6):638–44.
12. Ralph-Edwards A, Woo A, McCrindle BW, et al. Hypertrophic obstructive cardiomyopathy: comparison

of outcomes after myectomy or alcohol ablation adjusted by propensity score. J Thorac Cardiovasc Surg 2005;129(2):351–8.

13. Veselka J, Faber L, Liebregts M, et al. Outcome of alcohol septal ablation in mildly symptomatic patients with hypertrophic obstructive cardiomyopathy: a long-term follow-up study based on the Euro-Alcohol Septal Ablation Registry. J Am Heart Assoc 2017;6(5) [pii:e005735].

14. Jones BM, Krishnaswamy A, Smedira NG, et al. How symptomatic should a hypertrophic obstructive cardiomyopathy patient be to consider alcohol septal ablation? J Am Heart Assoc 2017;6(5) [pii:e006292].

15. Sorajja P, Nishimura RA, Gersh BJ, et al. Outcome of mildly symptomatic or asymptomatic obstructive hypertrophic cardiomyopathy: a long-term follow-up study. J Am Coll Cardiol 2009;54(3):234–41.

16. Sorajja P, Ommen SR, Holmes DR, et al. Survival after alcohol septal ablation for obstructive hypertrophic cardiomyopathy. Circulation 2012;126(20):2374–80.

17. Fifer MA, Baggish AL. Assessment of heart failure: invasive and noninvasive methods. In: Naidu S, editor. Hypertrophic cardiomyopathy. New York: Springer; 2015. p. 85–96.

18. McKay J, Nagueh SF. Alcohol septal ablation to reduce heart failure. Interv Cardiol Clin 2017;6(3):445–52.

19. Kitamura M, Amano Y, Takayama M, et al. Usefulness of non-anteroseptal region left ventricular hypertrophy using cardiac magnetic resonance to predict repeat alcohol septal ablation for refractory obstructive hypertrophic cardiomyopathy. Am J Cardiol 2017;120(1):124–30.

20. Lakkis N, Plana JC, Nagueh S, et al. Efficacy of nonsurgical septal reduction therapy in symptomatic patients with obstructive hypertrophic cardiomyopathy and provocable gradients. Am J Cardiol 2001;88(5):583–6.

21. Gietzen FH, Leuner CJ, Obergassel L, et al. Role of transcoronary ablation of septal hypertrophy in patients with hypertrophic cardiomyopathy, New York Heart Association functional class III or IV, and outflow obstruction only under provocable conditions. Circulation 2002;106(4):454–9.

22. Sigwart U. Non-surgical myocardial reduction for hypertrophic obstructive cardiomyopathy. Lancet 1995;346(8969):211–4.

23. Ayoub C, Geske JB, Larsen CM, et al. Comparison of Valsalva maneuver, amyl nitrite, and exercise echocardiography to demonstrate latent left ventricular outflow obstruction in hypertrophic cardiomyopathy. Am J Cardiol 2017;120(12):2265–71.

24. Kitamura M, Takayama M, Matsuda J, et al. Clinical characteristics and outcome of alcohol septal ablation with confirmation by nitroglycerin test for drug-refractory hypertrophic obstructive cardiomyopathy

with labile left ventricular outflow obstruction. Am J Cardiol 2015;116(6):945–51.

25. Prasad M, Geske JB, Sorajja P, et al. Hemodynamic changes in systolic and diastolic function during isoproterenol challenge predicts symptomatic response to myectomy in hypertrophic cardiomyopathy with labile obstruction. Catheter Cardiovasc Interv 2016;88(6):962–70.

26. Robbins RC, Stinson EB. Long-term results of left ventricular myotomy and myectomy for obstructive hypertrophic cardiomyopathy. J Thorac Cardiovasc Surg 1996;111(3):586–94.

27. Seggewiss H. Current status of alcohol septal ablation for patients with hypertrophic cardiomyopathy. Curr Cardiol Rep 2001;3(2):160–6.

28. Patel P, Dhillon A, Popovic ZB, et al. Left ventricular outflow tract obstruction in hypertrophic cardiomyopathy patients without severe septal hypertrophy: implications of mitral valve and papillary muscle abnormalities assessed using cardiac magnetic resonance and echocardiography. Circ Cardiovasc Imaging 2015;8(7):e003132.

29. Nishimura RA, Schaff HV. Evolving treatment for patients with hypertrophic obstructive cardiomyopathy. J Am Coll Cardiol 2015;66(15):1697–9.

30. Sorajja P, Pedersen WA, Bae R, et al. First experience with percutaneous mitral valve plication as primary therapy for symptomatic obstructive hypertrophic cardiomyopathy. J Am Coll Cardiol 2016;67(24):2811–8.

31. Veselka J, Duchonová R, Páleníčková J, et al. Age-related hemodynamic and morphologic differences in patients undergoing alcohol septal ablation for hypertrophic obstructive cardiomyopathy. Circ J 2006;70(7):880–4.

32. Liebregts M, Faber L, Jensen MK, et al. Outcomes of alcohol septal ablation in younger patients with obstructive hypertrophic cardiomyopathy. JACC Cardiovasc Interv 2017;10(11):1134–43.

33. Fifer MA. Septal ablation in younger patients: is it time to update the guidelines? JACC Cardiovasc Interv 2017;10(11):1144–6.

34. Lu M, Du H, Gao Z, et al. Predictors of outcome after alcohol septal ablation for hypertrophic obstructive cardiomyopathy: an echocardiography and cardiovascular magnetic resonance imaging study. Circ Cardiovasc Interv 2016;9(3):e002675.

35. Yang YJ, Fan CM, Yuan JQ, et al. Effectiveness of alcohol septal ablation in obstructive hypertrophic cardiomyopathy with versus without extreme septal hypertrophy. J Invasive Cardiol 2016;28(3):99–103.

36. Chen AA, Palacios IF, Mela T, et al. Acute predictors of subacute complete heart block after alcohol septal ablation for obstructive hypertrophic cardiomyopathy. Am J Cardiol 2006;97(2):264–9.

37. Talreja DR, Nishimura RA, Edwards WD, et al. Alcohol septal ablation versus surgical septal myectomy:

comparison of effects on atrioventricular conduction tissue. J Am Coll Cardiol 2004;44(12):2329–32.

38. Fifer MA, Sigwart U. Controversies in cardiovascular medicine. Hypertrophic obstructive cardiomyopathy: alcohol septal ablation. Eur Heart J 2011; 32(9):1059–64.

39. Qin JX, Shiota T, Lever HM, et al. Outcome of patients with hypertrophic obstructive cardiomyopathy after percutaneous transluminal septal myocardial ablation and septal myectomy surgery. J Am Coll Cardiol 2001;38(7):1994–2000.

40. Sorajja P, Valeti U, Nishimura RA, et al. Outcome of alcohol septal ablation for obstructive hypertrophic cardiomyopathy. Circulation 2008;118(2):131–9.

41. Ten Cate FJ, Soliman OII, Michels M, et al. Long-term outcome of alcohol septal ablation in patients with obstructive hypertrophic cardiomyopathy. A word of caution. Circ Heart Fail 2010;3(3):362–9.

42. Steggerda RC, Damman K, Balt JC, et al. Periprocedural complications and long-term outcome after alcohol septal ablation versus surgical myectomy in hypertrophic obstructive cardiomyopathy: a single-center experience. JACC Cardiovasc Interv 2014;7(11):1227–34.

43. Vriesendorp PA, Liebregts M, Steggerda RC, et al. Long-term outcomes after medical and invasive treatment in patients with hypertrophic cardiomyopathy. JACC Heart Fail 2014;2(6):630–6.

44. Agarwal S, Tuzcu EM, Desai MY, et al. Updated meta-analysis of septal alcohol ablation versus myectomy for hypertrophic cardiomyopathy. J Am Coll Cardiol 2010;55(8):823–34.

45. Leonardi RA, Kransdorf EP, Simel DL, et al. Meta-analyses of septal reduction therapies for obstructive hypertrophic cardiomyopathy: comparative rates of overall mortality and sudden cardiac death after treatment. Circ Cardiovasc Interv 2010;3(2):97–104.

46. Liebregts M, Vriesendorp PA, Mahmoodi BK, et al. A systematic review and meta-analysis of long-term outcomes after septal reduction therapy in patients with hypertrophic cardiomyopathy. JACC Heart Fail 2015;3(11):896–905.

47. Faber L, Seggewiss H, Gleichmann U. Percutaneous transluminal septal myocardial ablation in hypertrophic obstructive cardiomyopathy: results with respect to intraprocedural myocardial contrast echocardiography. Circulation 1998;98(22):2415–21.

48. Lakkis NM, Nagueh SF, Kleiman NS, et al. Echocardiography-guided ethanol septal reduction for hypertrophic obstructive cardiomyopathy. Circulation 1998;98(17):1750–5.

49. Sanborn DMY, Sigwart U, Fifer MA. Patient selection for alcohol septal ablation for hypertrophic obstructive cardiomyopathy: clinical and echocardiographic evaluation. Interv Cardiol 2012;4(3):349–59.

50. Kimmelstiel C. Reducing arrhythmic complications following alcohol septal ablation: the utility of lower doses of ethanol. Catheter Cardiovasc Interv 2010; 75(4):551–2.

51. Veselka J, Zemánek D, Tomasov P, et al. Complications of low-dose, echo-guided alcohol septal ablation. Catheter Cardiovasc Interv 2010;75(4):546–50.

52. Baggish AL, Smith RN, Palacios I, et al. Pathological effects of alcohol septal ablation for hypertrophic obstructive cardiomyopathy. Heart 2006;92(12): 1773–8.

53. Veselka J, Duchonová R, Procházková S, et al. The biphasic course of changes of left ventricular outflow gradient after alcohol septal ablation for hypertrophic obstructive cardiomyopathy. Kardiol Pol 2004; 60(2):133–6 [discussion: 137].

54. Yoerger DM, Picard MH, Palacios IF, et al. Time course of pressure gradient response after first alcohol septal ablation for obstructive hypertrophic cardiomyopathy. Am J Cardiol 2006;97(10):1511–4.

55. Schulz-Menger J, Strohm O, Waigand J, et al. The value of magnetic resonance imaging of the left ventricular outflow tract in patients with hypertrophic obstructive cardiomyopathy after septal artery embolization. Circulation 2000;101(15):1764–6.

56. Veselka J, Jensen MK, Liebregts M, et al. Long-term clinical outcome after alcohol septal ablation for obstructive hypertrophic cardiomyopathy: results from the Euro-ASA registry. Eur Heart J 2016; 37(19):1517–23.

57. van Dockum WG, Beek AM, ten Cate FJ, et al. Early onset and progression of left ventricular remodeling after alcohol septal ablation in hypertrophic obstructive cardiomyopathy. Circulation 2005;111(19):2503–8.

58. Chen YZ, Qiao SB, Hu FH, et al. Biventricular reverse remodeling after successful alcohol septal ablation for obstructive hypertrophic cardiomyopathy. Am J Cardiol 2015;115(4):493–8.

59. Matsuda J, Kitamura M, Takayama M, et al. Chronic phase improvements in electrocardiographic and echocardiographic manifestations of left ventricular hypertrophy after alcohol septal ablation for drug-refractory hypertrophic obstructive cardiomyopathy. Heart Vessels 2018;33(3):246–54.

60. Jassal DS, Neilan TG, Fifer MA, et al. Sustained improvement in left ventricular diastolic function after alcohol septal ablation for hypertrophic obstructive cardiomyopathy. Eur Heart J 2006;27(15): 1805–10.

61. Nagueh SF, Lakkis NM, Middleton KJ, et al. Changes in left ventricular filling and left atrial function six months after nonsurgical septal reduction therapy for hypertrophic obstructive cardiomyopathy. J Am Coll Cardiol 1999;34(4):1123–8.

62. Reinhard W, Ten Cate FJ, Scholten M, et al. Permanent pacing for complete atrioventricular block after nonsurgical (alcohol) septal reduction in patients with obstructive hypertrophic cardiomyopathy. Am J Cardiol 2004;93(8):1064–6.

63. Faber L, Welge D, Fassbender D, et al. Percutaneous septal ablation for symptomatic hypertrophic obstructive cardiomyopathy: managing the risk of procedure-related AV conduction disturbances. Int J Cardiol 2007;119(2):163–7.

64. Knight C, Sigwart U. Non-surgical ablation of the ventricular septum for the treatment of hypertrophic cardiomyopathy. Heart 1996;76(1):92.

65. Agarwal SC, Purcell IF, Furniss SS. Apical myocardial injury caused by collateralisation of a septal artery during ethanol septal ablation. Heart 2005; 91(1):e2.

66. Noseworthy PA, Rosenberg MA, Fifer MA, et al. Ventricular arrhythmia following alcohol septal ablation for obstructive hypertrophic cardiomyopathy. Am J Cardiol 2009;104(1):128–32.

67. Lakkis NM, Nagueh SF, Dunn JK, et al. Nonsurgical septal reduction therapy for hypertrophic obstructive cardiomyopathy: one-year follow-up. J Am Coll Cardiol 2000;36(3):852–5.

68. Rigopoulos AG, Daci S, Pfeiffer B, et al. Low occurrence of ventricular arrhythmias after alcohol septal ablation in high-risk patients with hypertrophic obstructive cardiomyopathy. Clin Res Cardiol 2016; 105(11):953–61.

69. Jensen MK, Prinz C, Horstkotte D, et al. Alcohol septal ablation in patients with hypertrophic obstructive cardiomyopathy: low incidence of sudden cardiac death and reduced risk profile. Heart 2013; 99(14):1012–7.

70. Liebregts M, Faber L, Jensen MK, et al. Validation of the HCM Risk-SCD model in patients with hypertrophic cardiomyopathy following alcohol septal ablation. Europace 2017. https://doi.org/10.1093/europace/eux251.

71. Veselka J, Krejčí J, Tomašov P, et al. Long-term survival after alcohol septal ablation for hypertrophic obstructive cardiomyopathy: a comparison with general population. Eur Heart J 2014;35(30):2040–5.

72. Cooper RM, Shahzad A, Newton J, et al. Intra-cardiac echocardiography in alcohol septal ablation: a prospective comparative study against transthoracic echocardiography. Echo Res Pract 2015; 2(1):9–17.

73. Yang YJ, Fan CM, Yuan JQ, et al. Effectiveness of alcohol septal ablation versus transaortic extended myectomy in hypertrophic cardiomyopathy with mid-ventricular obstruction. J Interv Cardiol 2016;29(6): 619–27.

74. Guerrero I, Dhoble A, Fasulo M, et al. Safety and efficacy of coil embolization of the septal perforator for septal ablation in patients with hypertrophic obstructive cardiomyopathy. Catheter Cardiovasc Interv 2016;88(6):971–7.

75. Shelke AB, Menon R, Kapadiya A, et al. A novel approach in the use of radiofrequency catheter ablation of septal hypertrophy in hypertrophic obstructive cardiomyopathy. Indian Heart J 2016; 68(5):618–23.

76. Keane D, Hynes B, King G, et al. Feasibility study of percutaneous transvalvular endomyocardial cryoablation for the treatment of hypertrophic obstructive cardiomyopathy. J Invasive Cardiol 2007;19(6): 247–51.

77. Krishnaswamy A, Tuzcu EM, Svensson LG, et al. Combined transcatheter aortic valve replacement and emergent alcohol septal ablation. Circulation 2013;128(18):e366–8.

78. Guerrero M, Wang DD, Himbert D, et al. Short-term results of alcohol septal ablation as a bail-out strategy to treat severe left ventricular outflow tract obstruction after transcatheter mitral valve replacement in patients with severe mitral annular calcification. Catheter Cardiovasc Interv 2017;90(7):1220–6.

Surgical Myectomy
Subaortic, Midventricular, and Apical

Anita Nguyen, MBBS, Hartzell V. Schaff, MD*

KEYWORDS

- Hypertrophic cardiomyopathy • Septal myectomy • Transaortic • Transapical

KEY POINTS

- Surgical septal myectomy is the gold standard treatment option for patients with hypertrophic cardiomyopathy whose symptoms do not respond to maximal medical management.
- Transaortic extended septal myectomy is used for patients with subaortic obstruction. In experienced centers, this surgical technique has excellent early operative mortality rates and long-term outcomes.
- For patients with apical hypertrophic cardiomyopathy or those with midventricular obstruction, a transapical incision may provide an alternative surgical approach.
- The combination of transaortic and transapical myectomy may be useful for patients with complex long-segment septal hypertrophy.

INTRODUCTION

The first operation for hypertrophic cardiomyopathy (HCM) was performed by Goodwin and colleagues[1] in 1958, and surgical management has evolved over the subsequent decades. Currently, the most widely performed operation for patients with subaortic obstruction is transaortic extended septal myectomy.[2,3] The outcomes achieved following extended septal myectomy performed in dedicated HCM centers should encourage clinicians to consider surgical referral of patients with medically refractory symptoms. Experienced teams report early 30-day mortality of 1% or less with a negligible risk of an iatrogenic ventricular septal defect.[4–6] Left ventricular outflow tract (LVOT) gradients are reliably relieved following surgery with durable improvement of symptoms.[7]

For patients with less common phenotypes of HCM, including those with midventricular obstruction and/or hypertrophy confined to the left ventricular (LV) apex, a transapical incision may provide better exposure. Although transapical myectomy is a unique procedure performed in few centers, early outcomes seem promising for patients with apical HCM and may be preferable to cardiac transplantation for those with advanced heart failure. The transapical approach also provides excellent exposure for myectomy in patients with midventricular obstruction.[8,9] And finally, transaortic and transapical myectomy can be combined in patients with complex long-segmental hypertrophy.[10]

In this article, we describe these surgical techniques and discuss important preoperative and postoperative considerations that may be pertinent to clinicians who treat patients with HCM.

PATIENT SELECTION AND PREOPERATIVE CONSIDERATIONS

Patient selection for operation is based on symptomatic status and imaging studies. Surgical management is usually reserved for patients who remain symptomatic despite maximal medical therapy or those patients who experience unacceptable side effects from medications. Drugs commonly used in patients with subaortic

Disclosure Statement: This work was supported by the Paul and Ruby Tsai Family.
Department of Cardiovascular Surgery, Mayo Clinic, 200 First Street Southwest, Rochester, MN 55905, USA
* Corresponding author.
E-mail address: schaff@mayo.edu

Cardiol Clin 37 (2019) 95–104
https://doi.org/10.1016/j.ccl.2018.08.006

obstruction include beta-blockers, calcium-channel blockers, and disopyramide.[11] In patients with midventricular obstruction or those with apical HCM, the role of medical management is less clear; however, beta-blockade or calcium-channel blockade may be tried as first-line therapy.[12]

Transthoracic Doppler echocardiography provides adequate information for surgical planning in most patients with subaortic LVOT obstruction. The study can quantify the LVOT gradient and document the presence of systolic anterior motion (SAM) and mitral valve regurgitation. If the resting LVOT gradient is minimal (<30 mm Hg), provoked maneuvers, such as Valsalva, inhalation of amyl nitrite, exercise, or infusion of isoproterenol should be performed. Some degree of mitral valve regurgitation is common in patients with obstructive HCM, and a posteriorly directed jet is usually associated with SAM. However, some clinicians wrongly assume that absence of a posteriorly directed jet indicates the presence of intrinsic mitral valve disease; the decision on mitral valve intervention should not be based on lack of this echocardiographic feature.

Septal morphology can also be visualized on transthoracic echocardiography, and basal septal thickness generally measures 20 to 22 mm. There is, however, a wide range of septal thickness in patients with subaortic obstruction. Indeed, some patients with obstructive HCM have relatively minor degrees of septal hypertrophy; but septal wall thickness should not be used as a contraindication to surgical myectomy, as outcomes are excellent in those with septal thickness less than 18 mm in experienced centers.[6]

In patients with midventricular obstruction, the gradient across the midventricle is also measured using Doppler echocardiography. However, for patients with hypertrophy confined to the LV apex (apical HCM), additional imaging studies, including cardiac MRI, may be necessary. Although Doppler echocardiography may visualize the small LV cavity, stroke volume can be estimated using cardiac MRI; transapical myectomy is only beneficial in patients with apical HCM whose stroke volume is reduced and can be enhanced by enlarging the LV cavity and end-diastolic volume. Apical aneurysms, which are usually seen in patients with midventricular obstruction and/or apical HCM, are best visualized using contrast echocardiography or cardiac MRI.[13]

SURGICAL TECHNIQUE
General Considerations

After induction of general anesthesia, we routinely perform transesophageal echocardiography to measure the LVOT gradient, systolic anterior motion, and mitral valve regurgitation. A median sternotomy provides the best exposure to the aorta and the LV, and is preferred over minimally invasive techniques. Before instituting cardiopulmonary bypass, we use direct needle manometry to measure the gradient between the aorta and the left ventricle. We routinely record both a resting gradient as well as a provoked gradient following a premature ventricular contraction, which is induced by gently tapping on the heart.[14]

We use central aortic cannulation and a 2-stage venous cannula in the right atrium to initiate cardiopulmonary bypass at normothermia. The aorta is then occluded, and the heart is arrested with antegrade cold blood cardioplegia. We usually infuse 1000 mL of cold blood cardioplegia because of increased LV mass in patients with obstructive HCM. A repeat infusion of 400 mL of cardioplegia is administered if the cross-clamp time extends beyond 20 minutes.

Subaortic Obstruction

As seen in **Fig. 1**, for patients with subaortic obstruction, we use an oblique incision in the aorta that extends into the noncoronary sinus 1 cm above the aortic annulus. This oblique aortotomy is important for adequate visualization of the subaortic area. Exposure can be enhanced by other maneuvers. First, pericardial stitches are used only on the right side in order to elevate the right side of the heart and allow the left ventricle to fall posteriorly. Second, the inferior edges of the aorta may be retracted using stay sutures. Third, a cardiotomy sucker is placed through the aortic valve at the commissure between the noncoronary and left aortic sinuses to retract the anterior leaflet of the mitral valve posteriorly. Finally, the operating table can be tilted toward the left to facilitate optimal alignment of the surgeon's view.

In most patients a white endocardial scar can be seen, which is the contact lesion produced by apposition of the septum and the anterior mitral valve leaflet; this lesion can serve as a guide to the length of the myectomy which must be extended apically beyond the contact lesion. We use a No. 10 knife blade on a long handle to begin the myectomy with an upward incision in the septum 3 to 4 mm to the right of the nadir of the right aortic sinus. Depth of myectomy is usually 8 mm (width of the No. 10 knife blade) and the incision is carried upwards toward the aortic annulus and then counterclockwise over to the attachment of the anterior leaflet of the mitral valve. Adequate extension of this incision toward the LV apex is

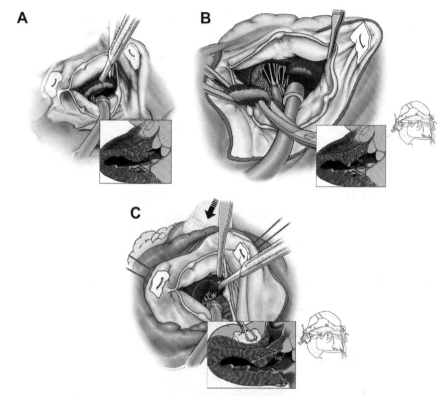

Fig. 1. Operative steps of septal myectomy with initial excision of the hypertrophied septum. The whitish endo-cardial scar is the point of contact between the anterior mitral valve leaflet and the septum (*A, B*). Panel (*C*) shows extension of the incision toward the apex of the LV. Arrow depicts a spongestick displacing the anterior wall of the left ventricle posteriorly to aid visualization. (*Courtesy of* Mayo Foundation for Medical Education and Research. All rights reserved; with permission.)

critically important as incomplete resection can lead to residual SAM and LVOT gradient. The method described earlier provides excellent relief of obstruction; in our experience, extension of septal excision medially (clockwise) is unneces-sary and may increase the risk of complete heart block.

Abnormal papillary muscles may be present and, if these insert into the body of the anterior leaflet of the mitral valve, may crowd the outflow tract contributing to obstruction (**Figs. 2** and **3**). These abnormal papillary muscles should be excised during the operation. However, anoma-lous muscle that inserts into the free edge of the

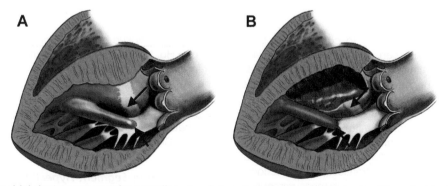

Fig. 2. Panel (*A*) depicts an anomalous papillary muscle inserting directly into the body of the mitral leaflet (*black arrows*). Panel (*B*) demonstrates insertion of an anomalous papillary muscle into the free edge of the anterior leaflet (*black arrows*); this does not contribute to obstruction and excision is not necessary. (*Courtesy of* Mayo Foundation for Medical Education and Research. All rights reserved; with permission.)

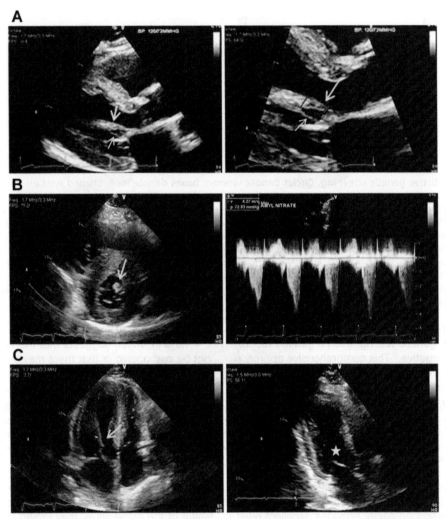

Fig. 3. Transthoracic echocardiogram demonstrating an anomalous papillary muscle inserting into the anterior mitral valve leaflet (*orange arrows* [*A*]). This papillary muscle contributes to LVOT obstruction (*yellow arrows* [*A–C*]). Panel (*A*) (*right side*) depicts the site of anomalous papillary muscle excision (*red lines*). Panel (*C*) (*right side*) shows results of septal myectomy and excision of the anomalous papillary muscle (*yellow star*) with preservation of chordal attachments to the leaflet edge. (*From* Kadkhodayan A, Schaff HV, Eleid MF. Anomalous papillary muscle insertion in hypertrophic cardiomyopathy. Eur Heart J Cardiovasc Imaging 2016;17(5):588; with permission.)

anterior leaflet is unlikely to contribute to LVOT obstruction and can be preserved. Similarly, chordal attachments from an anomalous papillary muscle to the free edge of the anterior leaflet should not be resected.[15]

Before closing the aortotomy, it is important to inspect both aortic and mitral valves for any inadvertent injury. The aorta is closed in 2 layers with a 4-0 polypropylene suture. Adequacy of operation is judged by postbypass transesophageal echocardiography and by direct pressure measurements. In most patients, there is no resting or provoked LVOT gradient. We would resume cardiopulmonary bypass and resect additional septal muscle if the

resting or provoked gradient is greater than 15 to 20 mm Hg. In some centers, isoproterenol infusion before and after myectomy may be used to serve the same purpose as direct pressure measurements, with gradients obtained via transesophageal echocardiography. Similarly, adequate myectomy eliminates SAM of the mitral leaflets, although chordal SAM may persist.

Complex Long-Segment Hypertrophy

In some patients, subaortic septal hypertrophy extends to the distal portion of the midventricle (complex long-segment hypertrophy) (**Fig. 4**).

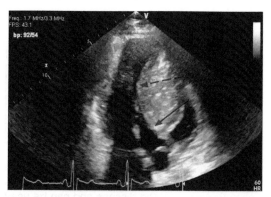

Fig. 4. Transthoracic echocardiogram of a patient with complex long-segment hypertrophy showing subaortic obstruction (*solid red arrow*) and midventricular obstruction (*dashed red arrow*). (*From* Hang D, Schaff HV, Ommen SR, et al. Combined transaortic and transapical approach to septal myectomy in patients with complex hypertrophic cardiomyopathy. J Thorac Cardiovasc Surg 2018;155(5):2097; with permission.)

Limiting the area of septal resection to the subaortic region may leave residual midventricular obstruction.[16] For these patients, we use a combined procedure, whereby muscle is resected proximally through the transaortic incision and distally through a transapical ventriculotomy (**Fig. 5**).[10]

We complete the transaortic myectomy as described earlier. Next, the apex of the heart is elevated anteriorly into view using 2 to 3 moist laparotomy pads. The incision into the apex is made starting to the left of the left anterior descending coronary artery and measures approximately 6 to 7 cm in length. It is important to incise the apex far enough lateral to the left anterior descending artery in order to avoid coronary injury during closure of the ventriculotomy. Septal muscle is excised from the midventricle and progresses proximally to join the subaortic resection. Often, there will be areas of endocardial scarring, which guide excision. Enlarged papillary muscles may also be shaved off during surgery. Following adequate resection to relieve obstruction at the midventricle, the ventriculotomy is closed linearly using a 2-layer approximation with a felt strip buttress.

Isolated Midventricular Obstruction

In patients with isolated midventricular obstruction, the mitral valve leaflets do not participate in the mechanism of obstruction (**Fig. 6**). These patients present with symptoms similar to those of patients with subaortic obstruction. Relief of the intraventricular gradient will improve and often

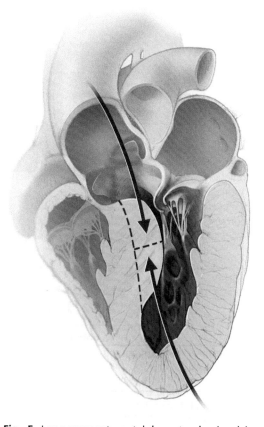

Fig. 5. Long-segment septal hypertrophy involving both the subaortic and midventricular regions is best managed using a combined transaortic (*red arrow and dashed lines*) and transapical approach (*blue arrow and dashed lines*). (*From* Hang D, Schaff HV, Ommen SR, et al. Combined transaortic and transapical approach to septal myectomy in patients with complex hypertrophic cardiomyopathy. J Thorac Cardiovasc Surg 2018;155(5):2097; with permission.)

eliminate associated dyspnea, angina, and syncope. Although some surgeons attempt midventricular myectomy through the aortic valve, we prefer exposure through the transapical incision, as seen in **Fig. 7**.[9]

Apical Hypertrophic Cardiomyopathy

Some patients with apical HCM have no subaortic or intraventricular gradients but develop symptoms of diastolic heart failure due to cavity obliteration and reduced stroke volume (**Fig. 8**A, B). In these patients, apical myectomy can be performed to enlarge the ventricular cavity, thereby augmenting LV end-diastolic volume and increasing stroke volume.

We perform a transapical myectomy by incising the LV apex, as described earlier (**Fig. 8**C, D). We

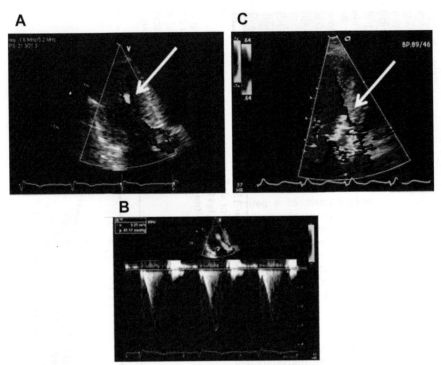

Fig. 6. Doppler echocardiography of a patient with midventricular obstruction. Panel (*A*) shows midventricular obstruction at the level of the papillary muscles (*white arrow*) without SAM of the mitral valve leaflet. Panel (*B*) shows the continuous-wave Doppler tracing at the midventricle. Panel (*C*) shows resolution of midventricular obstruction following transapical midventricular myectomy (*white arrow*). (*From* Kunkala MR, Schaff HV, Nishimura RA, et al. Transapical approach to myectomy for midventricular obstruction in hypertrophic cardiomyopathy. Ann Thorac Surg 2013;96(2):567; with permission.)

then identify and protect the anterolateral and posteromedial papillary muscles, and begin the myectomy on the ventricular septum to enlarge the LV cavity. If prominent papillary muscles are present, these may be shaved to further increase LV volume. The myectomy is extended proximally, beyond the midventricular level. Adequacy of muscle excision is judged visually and by palpation. The ventriculotomy is closed linearly, using Teflon felt buttress.

Apical Aneurysms

Apical aneurysms may occur in patients with apical HCM or those with midventricular obstruction due to high intraventricular pressure and subendocardial ischemia (**Fig. 9**). These aneurysms and associated endocardial scarring may contribute to ventricular arrhythmias and can also act as a site for thrombus formation leading to thromboembolic strokes. Thus, it is important to excise an apical aneurysm during transapical myectomy. The apical aneurysm is incised and resected completely. Careful resection of subendocardial scarring should also be performed. The defect is closed in 2 layers using polytetrafluoroethylene

(Teflon, The Chemours Company, Wilmington, DE) felt (**Fig. 10**).[13,17]

Postoperative Management

Following surgery, it is important to maintain high afterload; this can be achieved by using vasopressors to keep peripheral vascular resistance at an adequate level. Vasodilators should be avoided in the immediate postoperative period. We routinely use amiodarone prophylactically in most patients to avoid postoperative atrial fibrillation, as arrhythmias may be poorly tolerated by some patients. Conduction abnormalities are not uncommon postoperatively. Indeed, left bundle branch block is observed in up to 40% of patients following myectomy. But in our experience, only 3% of patients require permanent pacemaker insertion because of complete heart block.[6] Risk of complete heart block postoperatively is higher (35%) in those with preexisting right bundle branch block, which is often seen in patients who have previously undergone alcohol septal ablation.[18]

Before dismissal from the hospital, we routinely perform transthoracic echocardiography in all patients to determine the adequacy of LVOT gradient

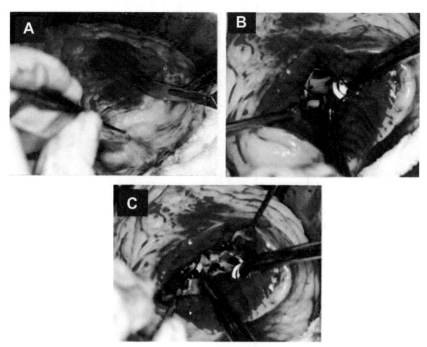

Fig. 7. Intraoperative photographs of a patient with midventricular obstruction who underwent transapical myectomy. Panel (*A*) shows the location of the incision. Panels (*B*) and (*C*) show the ventriculotomy. The endocardial scar can be seen on the anterolateral papillary muscle and the septum. (*From* Kunkala MR, Schaff HV, Nishimura RA, et al. Transapical approach to myectomy for midventricular obstruction in hypertrophic cardiomyopathy. Ann Thorac Surg 2013;96(2):566; with permission.)

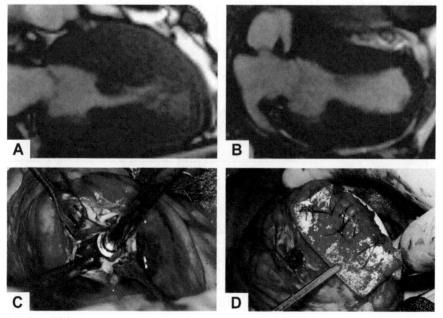

Fig. 8. Panels (*A*) and (*B*) are cardiac MRIs of a patient with apical HCM preoperatively (*A*) and after surgery (*B*). Panels (*C*) and (*D*) are intraoperative photographs showing surgical exposure (*C*) and closure of the ventriculotomy (*D*). (*From* Schaff HV, Brown ML, Dearani JA, et al. Apical myectomy: a new surgical technique for management of severely symptomatic patients with apical hypertrophic cardiomyopathy. J Thorac Cardiovasc Surg 2010;139(3):634–40; with permission.)

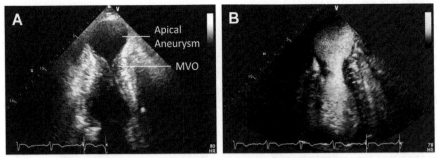

Fig. 9. Preoperative transthoracic echocardiogram of a patient with a large apical aneurysm and midventricular obstruction (MVO). Panel (*A*) shows the aneurysm and obstruction at the midventricular level. Panel (*B*) shows the same view with contrast, which is used to enhance visualization of apical aneurysms. (*From* Nguyen A, Schaff HV. Electrical storms in patients with apical aneurysms and hypertrophic cardiomyopathy with midventricular obstruction: a case series. J Thorac Cardiovasc Surg 2017;154(6):e102; with permission.)

relief and valvular function and assess for presence of a ventricular septal defect or pericardial effusion. Preoperative medications should be restarted before patient discharge, but some medications (eg, beta-blockers or disopyramide) may be prescribed at a lower dose or discontinued entirely.

OUTCOMES

Extended septal myectomy has excellent early outcomes for patients with subaortic obstruction, and operative mortality is less than 1% at experienced centers with dedicated HCM teams.[5] At the Mayo Clinic, we have performed transaortic

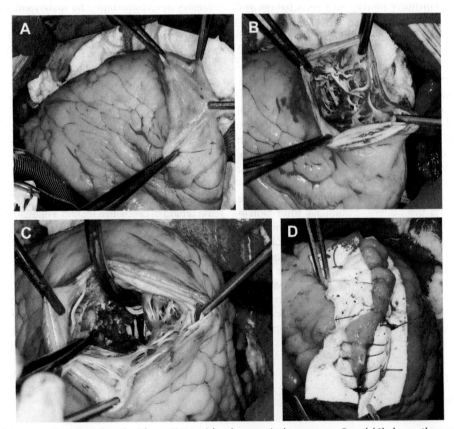

Fig. 10. Intraoperative photographs of a patient with a large apical aneurysm. Panel (*A*) shows the aneurysm at the LV apex. Panels (*B*) and (*C*) show the incised aneurysm and resection of hypertrophied muscle at the midventricular level. Panel (*D*) depicts the 2-layer closure of the ventriculotomy. (*From* Nguyen A, Schaff HV. Electrical storms in patients with apical aneurysms and hypertrophic cardiomyopathy with midventricular obstruction: a case series. J Thorac Cardiovasc Surg 2017;154(6):e102; with permission.)

extended septal myectomy in more than 3000 patients, with excellent short- and long-term outcomes. Complete relief of outflow tract gradient is achieved in most patients, and the complication of ventricular septal defect is rare (<1%) in our experience. Surgical results compare favorably with other septal reduction therapies, such as alcohol septal ablation, after which LVOT gradients may persist in some patients.[19]

Late survival following septal myectomy is excellent and, in some studies, comparable with an age- and sex-matched US population.[20] Indeed, survival of patients with obstructive HCM who undergo surgery seems significantly better than for those who are managed conservatively.[20] The primary indications for myectomy are limiting dyspnea, angina, or syncope; more than 90% of patients experience sustained reduction of their symptoms.[7] Inadequate symptomatic relief in patients with subaortic obstruction may be due to residual outflow tract obstruction; in most instances, this is the result of inadequate length of excision during initial myectomy.[16]

Extensive, long-segment septal hypertrophy presents a special problem because transaortic myectomy alone may be insufficient; residual septal hypertrophy in the midventricle can cause obstruction and lead to persistent symptoms. In such patients, we have performed combined transaortic and transapical septal myectomy. In these 86 patients, operative mortality was 2% and 1-year survival estimate was 95%.[10] Furthermore, symptomatic relief was excellent following the operation and 98% reported functional improvement at follow-up beyond 30 days.

We prefer a transapical approach for most patients with isolated midventricular obstruction, and Kunkala and colleagues[9] reported outcomes of 32 patients who underwent this procedure at our clinic. These investigators described 1- and 5-year survival estimates of 100% and 95%, and symptomatic status improved significantly following surgery (preoperative mean New York Heart Association [NYHA] class 2.9 ±0.7 vs postoperative mean NYHA class 1.3 ±0.6, $P<.001$). Importantly, there were no complications related to the apical incision reported in this series.

Similarly, early outcomes of transapical myectomy to enlarge LV end-diastolic volume in patients with apical HCM are encouraging; operative mortality has declined as surgeon experience has increased.[8] There has been no operative mortality following this procedure at our clinic since 2013. Furthermore, for patients with severe diastolic dysfunction due to apical HCM, the only alternative management is heart transplantation; transapical myectomy should be

considered before listing for heart transplantation. Indeed, informal comparisons of patients with apical HCM versus patients with HCM listed for heart transplantation show favorable survival in our surgical patients.

Patients with midventricular obstruction and concomitant apical aneurysms may present with thromboembolic complications and/or ventricular arrhythmias. Although conservative management is sufficient in some,[21] aneurysm resection and concomitant myectomy may be necessary for patients who have recurrent thromboembolism on anticoagulation, complications from anticoagulation, or persistent ventricular arrhythmias despite pharmacologic therapy. We have performed apical aneurysm resection in 44 patients with midventricular obstruction and/or apical HCM. Early outcomes are very encouraging, with no recurrent thromboembolic episodes and control of ventricular arrhythmias in 80% to 90% of patients following aneurysmectomy and myectomy.[13,17]

SUMMARY

HCM is a heterogeneous disease with multiple phenotypes and manifestations. Transaortic extended septal myectomy is the preferred treatment of most patients with subaortic obstruction whose symptoms are not alleviated with maximal medical therapy. A combined transaortic and transapical myectomy provides adequate exposure for patients with complex long-segmental HCM. For patients with midventricular obstruction or apical HCM, a transapical myectomy is a unique surgical management option. Apical aneurysms, which occur frequently in patients with midventricular obstruction or apical HCM, can also be resected and repaired using the transapical approach.

REFERENCES

1. Goodwin JF, Hollman A, Cleland WP, et al. Obstructive cardiomyopathy simulating aortic stenosis. Br Heart J 1960;22:403–14.
2. Messmer BJ. Extended myectomy for hypertrophic obstructive cardiomyopathy. Ann Thorac Surg 1994;58(2):575–7.
3. Nguyen A, Schaff HV. Transaortic septal myectomy for obstructive hypertrophic cardiomyopathy. Oper Tech Thorac Cardiovasc Surg 2018. https://doi.org/10.1053/j.optechstcvs.2018.06.001.
4. Maron BJ. Surgery for hypertrophic obstructive cardiomyopathy. Circulation 2005;111(16):2016–8.
5. Maron BJ, Dearani JA, Ommen SR, et al. Low operative mortality achieved with surgical septal

myectomy: role of dedicated hypertrophic cardio-myopathy centers in the management of dynamic subaortic obstruction. J Am Coll Cardiol 2015; 66(11):1307–8.

6. Nguyen A, Schaff HV, Nishimura RA, et al. Does septal thickness influence outcome of myectomy for hypertrophic obstructive cardiomyopathy? Eur J Cardiothorac Surg 2018;53(3):582–9.

7. Wells S, Rowin EJ, Boll G, et al. Clinical profile of nonresponders to surgical myectomy with obstructive hypertrophic cardiomyopathy. Am J Med 2018; 131(6):e235–9.

8. Schaff HV, Brown ML, Dearani JA, et al. Apical myectomy: a new surgical technique for management of severely symptomatic patients with apical hypertrophic cardiomyopathy. J Thorac Cardiovasc Surg 2010;139(3):634–40.

9. Kunkala MR, Schaff HV, Nishimura RA, et al. Transapical approach to myectomy for midventricular obstruction in hypertrophic cardiomyopathy. Ann Thorac Surg 2013;96(2):564–70.

10. Hang D, Schaff HV, Ommen SR, et al. Combined transaortic and transapical approach to septal myectomy in patients with complex hypertrophic cardiomyopathy. J Thorac Cardiovasc Surg 2018; 155(5):2096–102.

11. Gersh BJ, Maron BJ, Bonow RO, et al. 2011 ACCF/AHA guideline for the diagnosis and treatment of hypertrophic cardiomyopathy: a report of the American College of Cardiology Foundation/American Heart Association Task Force on Practice Guidelines. Circulation 2011;124(24):e783–831.

12. Jan MF, Todaro MC, Oreto L, et al. Apical hypertrophic cardiomyopathy: present status. Int J Cardiol 2016;222:745–59.

13. Nguyen A, Schaff HV, Nishimura RA, et al. Early outcomes of repair of left ventricular apical aneurysms in patients with hypertrophic cardiomyopathy. Circulation 2017;136(20):1979–81.

14. Trevino AR, Buergler J. The Brockenbrough-Braunwald-Morrow sign. Methodist Debakey Cardiovasc J 2014;10(1):34–7.

15. Kadkhodayan A, Schaff HV, Eleid MF. Anomalous papillary muscle insertion in hypertrophic cardiomyopathy. Eur Heart J Cardiovasc Imaging 2016;17(5):588.

16. Cho YH, Quintana E, Schaff HV, et al. Residual and recurrent gradients after septal myectomy for hypertrophic cardiomyopathy-mechanisms of obstruction and outcomes of reoperation. J Thorac Cardiovasc Surg 2014;148(3):909–15 [discussion: 915–6].

17. Nguyen A, Schaff HV. Electrical storms in patients with apical aneurysms and hypertrophic cardiomyopathy with midventricular obstruction: a case series. J Thorac Cardiovasc Surg 2017;154(6):e101–3.

18. Talreja DR, Nishimura RA, Edwards WD, et al. Alcohol septal ablation versus surgical septal myectomy: comparison of effects on atrioventricular conduction tissue. J Am Coll Cardiol 2004;44(12): 2329–32.

19. Sorajja P, Ommen SR, Holmes DR Jr, et al. Survival after alcohol septal ablation for obstructive hypertrophic cardiomyopathy. Circulation 2012;126(20): 2374–80.

20. Ommen SR, Maron BJ, Olivotto I, et al. Long-term effects of surgical septal myectomy on survival in patients with obstructive hypertrophic cardiomyopathy. J Am Coll Cardiol 2005;46(3):470–6.

21. Rowin EJ, Maron BJ, Haas TS, et al. Hypertrophic cardiomyopathy with left ventricular apical aneurysm: implications for risk stratification and management. J Am Coll Cardiol 2017;69(7):761–73.

Advanced Heart Failure Management and Transplantation

Avi Levine, MD[a],*, Chhaya Aggarwal Gupta, MD[a],
Alan Gass, MD[b]

KEYWORDS

- Hypertrophic cardiomyopathy • Heart failure • LVAD • Cardiac transplant

KEY POINTS

- Hypertrophic cardiomyopathy (HCM) is a genetic heart disease with heterogeneous clinical features, including progression to advanced heart failure.
- Development of advanced heart failure symptoms can be related to outflow obstruction but in some patients reflects an underlying process of fibrosis and progressive ventricular dysfunction.
- Left ventricular assist device support is infrequently used due to the restrictive physiology underlying HCM, but cardiac transplantation represents an effective treatment, with encouraging long-term outcome data.

INTRODUCTION

Hypertrophic cardiomyopathy (HCM) is the most common genetic heart disease, with a heterogeneous expression of clinical, morphologic, and functional features.[1] One of the most recognized and tragic complications of HCM is sudden cardiac death (SCD). With the development of risk stratification models and increased use of implantable cardioverter-defibrillators, the rates of SCD have declined significantly.[2,3] This reduction in SCD has resulted in a greater focus on myocardial dysfunction associated with the disease leading to the development of clinical heart failure.[4] There is a subset of HCM patients who progress to advanced heart failure, characterized by New York Heart Association (NYHA) functional classes III and IV. This review focuses on the pathophysiology of advanced heart failure in HCM as well as management options for end-stage disease, including mechanical circulatory support and cardiac transplantation.

ADVANCED HEART FAILURE

Heart failure represents a complex clinical syndrome marked by signs and symptoms of the heart's inability to deliver appropriate flow to the other organs. Within the realm of HCM, there are 2 types of phenotypes in patients who develop heart failure symptoms: obstructive and nonobstructive.[4]

Hypertrophic Cardiomyopathy with Obstruction

The more common cause of heart failure symptoms in the HCM population is related to flow

Disclosure Statement: A. Gass—Speaker's Bureau, Medtronic, Abbott Vascular. All other authors have no relevant disclosures.
[a] Advanced Heart Failure and Cardiac Transplantation, Division of Cardiology, Department of Medicine, Westchester Medical Center, New York Medical College, Macy Pavilion, Suite 100, 100 Woods Road, Valhalla, NY 10595, USA; [b] Heart Transplant and Mechanical Circulatory Support, Division of Cardiology, Department of Medicine, Westchester Medical Center, New York Medical College, Macy Pavilion, Suite 100, 100 Woods Road, Valhalla, NY 10595, USA
* Corresponding author.
E-mail address: elliot.levine@wmchealth.org

Cardiol Clin 37 (2019) 105–111
https://doi.org/10.1016/j.ccl.2018.08.007

obstruction. With ventricular hypertrophy, the left ventricular (LV) cavity size is reduced and is accompanied by LV outflow obstruction in the setting of preserved or even hyperdynamic LV function. This leads to an increase in filling pressures, a reduction in cardiac output, and myocardial demand ischemia. Furthermore, there can be mitral valve abnormalities, including systolic anterior motion of the leaflet apparatus or primary valvular pathology related to the HCM disease process itself, leading to mitral regurgitation and worsening of the heart failure cascade. The resulting symptoms of shortness of breath and fatigue can be with exertion or even present at rest.

There are several management strategies for outflow obstruction. Medical therapy includes negative inotropic agents, such as β-blockers, calcium channel blockers, or even antiarrhythmic agents, such as disopyramide. Diuretic dose is usually lowered or discontinued to allow for greater LV filling, reducing the degree of obstruction. Beyond pharmacologic options, there are mechanical septal reduction strategies that include alcohol septal ablation and surgical myectomy.

Nonobstructive Hypertrophic Cardiomyopathy

On the other end of the HCM spectrum, there is a subset of patients with nonobstructive physiology who may progress to severe functional limitation refractory to maximal medical management, termed end-stage or burnt-out HCM.

Pathophysiology

Within the nonobstructive subgroup, there are multiple distinct phenotypes: (1) mild hypertrophy or even regression of septal thickness, with replacement fibrosis and ventricular remodeling leading to LV cavity enlargement and systolic impairment; (2) preserved hypertrophy with LV cavity enlargement; (3) normal LV cavity size and only minimal increase in hypertrophy (<20 mm); and (4) marked hypertrophy (20–39 mm) with a nondilated ventricle.[5]

Myocardial fibrosis is the dominant pathophysiologic abnormality underlying this advanced disease process. The development of fibrosis is part of the phenotypic expression of HCM but also may be related to abnormal intramural coronary arteries, which produce ischemia and ultimately fibrosis.[6] Autopsy data from explanted hearts at the time of transplant have provided insight into the histologic basis of the fibrotic disease process.[7] Three different fibrosis types have been identified: interstitial perimyocyte, mixed fibrosis, and replacement (scarlike) fibrosis, with replacement fibrosis representing the most prevalent type. Fibrosis is most extensive in the midwall of the ventricle, preferentially involves the apex of the heart, and only marginally involves the right ventricle. A correlation between degree of fibrosis and degree of ventricular dilatation has been reported in the pathology literature.[8]

There have also been certain genotypic features associated with the development of ventricular dysfunction. Certain genetic mutations have been linked to heart failure endpoints and end-stage HCM, specifically involving the myosin heavy chain and myosin-binding proteins.[9–11] Whether a different screening or treatment approach should be used for patients with these mutations, however, remains unknown.

Clinical burden

Progression to advanced heart failure symptoms within the nonobstructive HCM group seems less frequent than in those patients with obstruction.[12] The incidence of advanced disease unrelated to outflow obstruction has been estimated at 3% to 10%,[4,5,12,13] with a reported rate of annual progression to NYHA III/IV symptoms of 1.6% per year.[12] In general, end-stage HCM represents a more aggressive phenotype, with diagnosis at an earlier age,[5] and it carries high morbidity and mortality. In a large study from London, 5-year survival free from death, implantable cardioverter-defibrillator discharge, or transplant was only 52% for end-stage HCM versus 90% in other HCM patients.[14] Survival alone is significantly decreased at 1 year and 5 years after diagnosis,[8] and a large study from Italy has demonstrated approximately 50% mortality at 6 years.[13] Although the time from initial diagnosis of HCM to development of end-stage disease can be prolonged, with studies showing ranges of 8 years to 14 years,[5,13] the time from end-stage HCM diagnosis until death or transplant is much shorter, approximately 2.7 years.[5]

Although a small minority of HCM patients initially present with advanced nonobstructive disease, most patients develop symptom progression over time. In 1 study looking at paired echocardiograms, LV end-diastolic dimension (LVEDD) increased at a rate of 1.7 mm per year, although septal thickness decreased at a rate of 1.4 mm per year. At the same time, on average, LV ejection fraction (LVEF) decreased by 6.1% per year. For patients with an initially normal LVEF, yearly incidence of systolic impairment has been estimated at 0.87%.[14]

Noninvasive imaging

Noninvasive imaging can be valuable in the evaluation of HCM patients with progressive heart failure. Cardiac MRI has many applications within the realm of HCM, and the presence of late gadolinium enhancement (LGE) has been particularly useful for heart failure endpoints. In 1 study looking at HCM patients with nonobstructive physiology, more extensive LGE correlated with risk of progression to NYHA III/IV symptoms.[12] In another study, a multivariate analysis looking at parameters that include age, LV outflow gradient, and left atrial parameters demonstrated LGE was the only predictor of systolic dysfunction.[15] In this study, the analysis also exhibited a strong inverse correlation between the percentage of myocardium occupied by LGE and LVEF.[15]

Another heavily used noninvasive tool in the work-up and management of advanced heart failure is cardiopulmonary exercise testing (CPET). In systolic heart failure, both low peak oxygen consumption (Vo_2) and high minute ventilation/carbon dioxide production (VE/VCO2) slope a marker for ventilatory insufficiency, have proved prognostic markers for adverse outcomes and are used to guide timing for advanced therapies, such as cardiac transplantation.[16] In diastolic heart failure, distinct physiologically from systolic dysfunction, 1 large study suggested only VE/Vco_2 slope as a proved prognostic marker for a combined endpoint, including mortality and heart failure hospitalization.[17] Multiple studies looking at CPET results specifically for the HCM population have shown, however, that both peak Vo_2 and VE/Vco_2 slope are valid prognostic markers.[18,19] It was estimated that for HCM patients, the risk of death or transplant was reduced by 21% for every 1-mL/kg/min increase in peak Vo_2 and increased by 18% for each 1-unit increase in VE/Vco_2 slope. CPET parameters can be used to identify patients at high risk for disease progression and early mortality from heart failure events within the realm of HCM.

Pharmacologic treatment

In heart failure with reduced ejection fraction, the mainstay of guideline-directed medical therapy relies on neurohormonal blockade of the renin-angiotensin-aldosterone system (RAAS) and sympathetic nervous system. This includes β-blockers, angiotensin-converting enzyme inhibitors, angiotensin receptor blockers, angiotensin receptor–neprilysin inhibitors, and mineralocorticoid aldosterone antagonists.[20] Neurohormonal blockade, however, has not been rigorously studies within the HCM population. A recent small study investigated the effect of spironolactone on myocardial fibrosis and heart failure clinical endpoints in HCM, but no benefit was identified.[21] Nonetheless, for HCM patients with systolic

dysfunction, it is recommended to initiate these guideline-directed medical therapy medications when the ejection fraction drops below 50%, based on the data available for the general heart failure population. This recommendation has been given a class I indication, according to the 2011 American College of Cardiology Foundation/American Heart Association HCM guidelines, and a class IIa indication, according to the 2014 European Society of Cardiology HCM guidelines.[3,22]

Cardiac resynchronization therapy

For patients with systolic heart failure and evidence of electrical dyssynchrony on electrocardiogram, biventricular pacing or cardiac resynchronization therapy (CRT) is an established treatment modality that can help improve cardiac contractile function, heart failure symptoms, and mortality.[3,23,24] In HCM, electromechanical dyssynchrony has been linked to endpoints such as SCD.[25] Small retrospective studies, however, have not shown clear benefit for CRT use in patients with end-stage HCM and abnormal ventricular conduction.[26] Although a minority of these patients experienced improvement in NYHA class, overall there was no change in ejection fraction. This may be related to the unique pathophysiology of the underlying disease process, because electrical resynchronization is not expected to reverse underlying fibrosis.

Atrial fibrillation

Atrial fibrillation (AF) is the most common sustained arrhythmia in HCM, affecting approximately 20% of patients, and can lead to worsening of clinical symptoms.[27] This arrhythmia is related to diastolic dysfunction, left atrial enlargement, and remodeling as well as myocardial fibrosis and ischemia. HCM patients with AF tend to be older, have higher brain natriuretic peptide levels, and have a higher prevalence of coronary artery disease or prior stroke.[27] From a hemodynamic standpoint, in HCM, with abnormal diastolic function, the loss of atrial contraction and atrioventricular synchrony that occurs with AF can cause a significant decline in cardiac output. This leads to development of worsening heart failure symptoms and has even been associated with an increased risk of mortality unrelated to SCD.[27]

Treatment of AF is important for prevention of worsening heart failure symptoms. Acute episodes of AF can be treated with electrical or pharmacologic cardioversion, and antiarrhythmic medications or even AF ablation can be used to prevent AF recurrence. Beyond treatment strategies, prevention of AF would likely avert significant morbidity in HCM. The RAAS system has been implicated in atrial electrical remodeling and structural transformation.[28] Post hoc analysis of large trials for patients with coronary artery disease has suggested that RAAS inhibition, specifically angiotensin receptor blockade therapy, might reduce the onset of new AF.[29] For HCM specifically, a large retrospective study from Taiwan showed a reduced risk of AF development for HCM patients taking RAAS-inhibiting medications.[30] Further trials would be required to determine whether RAAS inhibition should be used as a primary prevention strategy for AF.

ADVANCED THERAPIES IN HYPERTROPHIC CARDIOMYOPATHY

Once patients have developed end-stage HCM, there are no effective medical options to halt or reverse disease progression, and advanced therapies should be considered. These include LV assist devices (LVADs) and cardiac transplantation.

Left Ventricular Assist Device

LVAD support is a form of mechanical circulatory support (MCS) used for advanced heart failure. The current generation of LVAD technology features a centrifugal flow pump that transports blood from an inflow cannula attached to the LV through an outflow graft leading to the arterial system, in essence bypassing the function of a failing heart.

There are many challenges to the implantation of LVAD support in HCM patients. First, despite LVAD support, there is still ongoing impaired diastolic filling, the primary pathophysiologic disease mechanism underlying symptom progression. In addition, HCM patients have a small cavity size and there is concern for suck-down events, perhaps even precipitating ventricular arrhythmias in a population at higher baseline risk for SCD. Moreover, the LVAD can contribute to right ventricular failure via various mechanisms, including shifting of the interventricular septum or creation of a hemodynamic burden to support LVAD flow. Nonetheless, there is clinical experience with LVAD support in HCM, and it may represent a viable option for certain patients.

HCM patients represent a very small percentage of patients on LVAD support. An analysis of INTERMACS (Interagency Registry for Mechanically Assisted Circulatory Support) data from 2008 to 2014, which included 9689 patients who received LVAD support, showed only 94 patients (0.9%) had an established diagnosis of HCM.[31] In comparison to patients with dilated cardiomyopathy (DCM), HCM patients tended to be younger (51.8 years old vs 57 years old), had a smaller LVEDD (6.1 vs 6.9 cm), and had higher LVEF. Only 4.8% of the LVAD HCM population had LVEF greater than 40%, so the HCM group on LVAD support likely represents a subset of patients with a mixed phenotype sharing many characteristics with DCM.[31]

Outcomes do not seem to be impaired for HCM patients on LVAD support. In a smaller series from the Mayo Clinic from 2007 to 2010, only 4.8% of all LVAD implants were patients with HCM or restrictive cardiomyopathy (RCM).[32] These patients had smaller LV cavities, thicker septal walls, and higher ejection fractions and were mostly implanted as bridge-to-transplant intention. Although patients in the HCM/RCM group trended toward more prolonged duration of postoperative inotropic support, higher infection rate, lower cardiac output after implant, and higher postoperative RA pressures, there was no difference in early or 1-year mortality compared with patients with DCM.

From a surgical standpoint, there have even been nonconventional strategies used to allow for LVAD implantation in HCM patients. In the series from the Mayo Clinic, there was a report of myomectomy to allow for placement of the inflow cannula at the time of LVAD implantation.[32] There is even a case report of left atrial cannulation via a right atrial approach to allow for LVAD implantation in an HCM patient with a small ventricular cavity.[33]

Cardiac Transplantation

Cardiac transplantation represents an effective long-term treatment of all end-stage heart failure patients, including end-stage HCM. HCM patients should represent ideal transplant candidates, because patients tend to manifest with advanced disease at an earlier age given HCM's genetic basis. In general, younger age translates into fewer major comorbidities, including significant atherosclerotic and renal disease that can lead to adverse outcomes after transplant. One important variable for obstructive HCM patients with prior septal reduction surgery and transfusions, however, is the possibility that they can have higher levels of antibodies, thereby restricting the potential donor pool.

The ability for HCM patients to receive an organ may be limited by the current listing system. The United Network for Organ Sharing (UNOS) has established levels of priority for patients awaiting transplant based on clinical condition to create fairness in allocation of organs to patients with the highest risk of death. Status 2 patients are the most stable, whereas status 1 represents patients in more immediate need of transplant.

Status 1 is further subdivided into status 1B, usually patients on stable LVAD support or intravenous inotropes, and status 1A, the highest level of urgency, for patients requiring continuous hemodynamic monitoring or mechanical support, such as intra-aortic balloon pump or extracorporeal membrane oxygenation. Because HCM patients, especially those without LV dilation or LV dysfunction, do not generally benefit from inotropic or mechanical support given the unique physiology, they usually remain status 2 or require UNOS exception for their status to be upgraded. This can extend wait-list time or even preclude transplant for patients in regions of the country with long wait-list times, because the overwhelming majority of transplants are transplanted as status 1A.

This barrier to transplant for HCM patients has been an active discussion point as the heart transplant community prepares to move to a new heart allocation system. Expected to be initiated in late 2018, the new system was in part developed to establish higher priority levels for patients with RCM or HCM. There are 6 tiers, with tier 1 representing the highest level of urgency for transplant. Under the new allocation scheme, patients with hypertrophic or RCM would be assigned tier 4. Given the persistent limitations this tier system places on the ability of HCM patients to receive a transplant, there is currently a proposal in the public comment phase at the time of publication of this article that suggests recommended criteria by which patients with HCM/RCM can be upgraded to tier 2 or tier 3. These criteria include hemodynamic monitoring and inotrope use as well as markers of hemodynamic instability and end-organ dysfunction.

UNOS data from 2006 to 2016 showed that of 30,608 patients placed on the wait list within the United States, 1562 (5.1%) carried a diagnosis of HCM or RCM.[34] In a separate analysis limited to HCM patients, the wait-list data from the Scientific Registry of Transplant Recipients (SRTR) were divided into 2 periods: 1999 to 2008 and 2008 to 2016.[35] Compared with the earlier period, the percentage of HCM patients in the later period increased from 1.6% to 2.3% ($P = .04$). Another unique feature that emerges from the SRTR data is the criteria used for listing status among HCM patients. For listing indications that fall outside the scope of standardized transplant urgency criteria, transplant centers are able to request consideration from the regional review board for status upgrade by exception criteria. Overall rates of patients upgraded to status 1A or status 1B by exception have increased across all cardiomyopathy groups from the earlier to the later period. The

increase among HCM patients, however, has been significantly more pronounced.

Analysis of these databases also provides insight into the difference in wait-list characteristics for patients with HCM.[34,35] Compared with DCM, HCM patients are younger, have a higher relative female percentage, and tend to have less major comorbidities, such as diabetes mellitus. In addition, consistent with the underlying restrictive physiology, the utilization of MCS is significantly lower in the HCM/RCM group (16.3 vs 42.8%). There is a higher utilization of MCS among HCM/RCM patients listed status 1A (39.5%) versus HCM/RCM patients with other statuses, perhaps reflecting a disease phenotype with a remodeled and dilated LV, but that percentage is still significantly lower than DCM patients listed status 1A (62.6%). In regard to duration of wait-list time, despite the barriers to transplant described previously, HCM/RCM patients experience a shorter overall average wait-list time (262.5 vs 293.6 days), with an average of 56.2 days fewer for the group of patients listed status 1A, and have a slightly higher incidence of transplant off the wait-list.

Outcome data have been favorable for HCM patients on the wait-list. Despite data showing increased wait-list mortality for certain subsets of patients, including congenital heart disease and those with prior transplant, multiple studies have demonstrated no difference in wait-list mortality or rate of delisting between HCM and DCM patients.[34–36] The only negative outcome that seems increased in HCM patients on the wait list is a higher rate of decline in functional status from the time of listing to the time of transplant.[35] Standard predictors of survival on the wait list, including age, body mass index, stroke, diabetes, and LVAD support, do not predict outcome for HCM patients. Instead, markers of functional status, frailty, renal function, and elevated filling pressures and the use of inotropes have proved valid predictors of wait-list mortality for HCM patients.

Most importantly, survival post-transplant is encouraging for HCM patients. There have been concerns that, in patients with HCM with restrictive physiology and elevated filling pressures, higher pulmonary pressures can lead to greater risk of right ventricular failure after transplant, thereby having an impact on survival. Nonetheless, survival after transplant seems equivalent, if not better, for HCM patients compared with other groups.[13,34,35,37] Looking at the UNOS database, from 1990 to 2004, of the 26,706 patients who underwent heart-only transplant, 303 patients, or 1%, had a diagnosis of HCM. The 1-year, 5-year, and 10-year overall survival rates after transplant were 85%, 75%, and 61%, respectively, for HCM patients. This trended toward greater survival compared with all non-HCM patients, who showed survival rates of 82%, 70%, and 49%, respectively (P = .05).[37] More recent data show perhaps even better transplant outcomes for HCM, especially long-term survival. Looking at the SRTR data for 2000 to 2016, the 5-year survival rate among HCM patients is 82.5%, significantly higher than other groups, with survival curves separating after 1 year.[35] In either analysis, when the non-HCM group is further subdivided into DCM versus ischemic cardiomyopathy, studies demonstrate a significantly greater survival for HCM patients versus those with ischemic cardiomyopathy at all intervals.[35,37]

One theoretic concern after transplant for HCM patients is the recurrence of hypertrophic pathology in the transplanted heart, including LV hypertrophy or fibrosis. This is especially relevant given the genetic basis of the disease and the young age at which many patients are transplanted. The majority of post-transplant analysis for HCM has focused on survival data, but 1 single-center HCM experience showed no recurrence of disease on routine post-transplant endomyocardial biopsies.[38]

SUMMARY

HCM is a genetic heart disease with heterogeneous clinical features, including progression to advanced heart failure. The development of these symptoms can be related to mechanical outflow obstruction but in some patients reflects an underlying process of fibrosis and progressive LV dysfunction. For these patients with end-stage disease, traditional heart failure therapies, including neurohormonal blockade or even CRT therapy, have not proved beneficial. As such, more advanced therapies, such as LVAD or cardiac transplantation, should be considered for these patients. Although LVAD support is infrequently used due to the restrictive physiology underlying HCM, transplant represents an effective treatment, with encouraging long-term outcome data.

REFERENCES

1. Maron BJ, Ommen SR, Semsarian C, et al. Hypertrophic cardiomyopathy: present and future, with translation into contemporary cardiovascular medicine. J Am Coll Cardiol 2014;64(1):83–99.
2. Maron BJ, Spirito P, Shen WK, et al. Implantable cardioverter-defibrillators and prevention of sudden cardiac death in hypertrophic cardiomyopathy. JAMA 2007;298(4):405–12.
3. Gersh BJ, Maron BJ, Bonow RO, et al. 2011 ACCF/AHA guideline for the diagnosis and treatment of hypertrophic cardiomyopathy: executive summary: a report of the American College of Cardiology Foundation/American Heart Association Task Force on practice guidelines. J Thorac Cardiovasc Surg 2011;142(6):1303–38.
4. Maron BJ, Rowin EJ, Udelson JE, et al. Clinical spectrum and management of heart failure in hypertrophic cardiomyopathy. JACC Heart Fail 2018;6(5):353–63.
5. Harris KM, Spirito P, Maron MS, et al. Prevalence, clinical profile, and significance of left ventricular remodeling in the end-stage phase of hypertrophic cardiomyopathy. Circulation 2006;114(3):216–25.
6. Maron BJ, Wolfson JK, Epstein SE, et al. Intramural ("small vessel") coronary artery disease in hypertrophic cardiomyopathy. J Am Coll Cardiol 1986;8(3):545–57.
7. Galati G, Leone O, Pasquale F, et al. Histological and histometric characterization of myocardial fibrosis in end-stage hypertrophic cardiomyopathy: a clinical-pathological study of 30 explanted hearts. Circ Heart Fail 2016;9(9) [pii:e003090].
8. Fernandez A, Vigliano CA, Casabe JH, et al. Comparison of prevalence, clinical course, and pathological findings of left ventricular systolic impairment versus normal systolic function in patients with hypertrophic cardiomyopathy. Am J Cardiol 2011;108(4):548–55.
9. Fujino N, Shimizu M, Ino H, et al. Cardiac troponin T Arg92Trp mutation and progression from hypertrophic to dilated cardiomyopathy. Clin Cardiol 2001;24(5):397–402.
10. Fujino N, Shimizu M, Ino H, et al. A novel mutation Lys273Glu in the cardiac troponin T gene shows high degree of penetrance and transition from hypertrophic to dilated cardiomyopathy. Am J Cardiol 2002;89(1):29–33.
11. Li Q, Gruner C, Chan RH, et al. Genotype-positive status in patients with hypertrophic cardiomyopathy is associated with higher rates of heart failure events. Circ Cardiovasc Genet 2014;7(4):416–22.
12. Maron MS, Rowin EJ, Olivotto I, et al. Contemporary natural history and management of nonobstructive hypertrophic cardiomyopathy. J Am Coll Cardiol 2016;67(12):1399–409.
13. Pasqualucci D, Fornaro A, Castelli G, et al. Clinical spectrum, therapeutic options, and outcome of advanced heart failure in hypertrophic cardiomyopathy. Circ Heart Fail 2015;8(6):1014–21.
14. Thaman R, Gimeno JR, Murphy RT, et al. Prevalence and clinical significance of systolic impairment in hypertrophic cardiomyopathy. Heart 2005;91(7):920–5.
15. Olivotto I, Maron BJ, Appelbaum E, et al. Spectrum and clinical significance of systolic function and

myocardial fibrosis assessed by cardiovascular magnetic resonance in hypertrophic cardiomyopathy. Am J Cardiol 2010;106(2):261–7.

16. Mancini DM, Eisen H, Kussmaul W, et al. Value of peak exercise oxygen consumption for optimal timing of cardiac transplantation in ambulatory patients with heart failure. Circulation 1991;83(3):778–86.

17. Guazzi M, Myers J, Arena R. Cardiopulmonary exercise testing in the clinical and prognostic assessment of diastolic heart failure. J Am Coll Cardiol 2005;46(10):1883–90.

18. Finocchiaro G, Haddad F, Knowles JW, et al. Cardiopulmonary responses and prognosis in hypertrophic cardiomyopathy: a potential role for comprehensive noninvasive hemodynamic assessment. JACC Heart Fail 2015;3(5):408–18.

19. Coats CJ, Rantell K, Bartnik A, et al. Cardiopulmonary exercise testing and prognosis in hypertrophic cardiomyopathy. Circ Heart Fail 2015;8(6):1022–31.

20. Yancy CW, Jessup M, Bozkurt B, et al. 2017 ACC/AHA/HFSA focused update of the 2013 ACCF/AHA guideline for the management of heart failure: a report of the American College of Cardiology/American Heart Association Task Force on clinical practice guidelines and the Heart Failure Society of America. J Am Coll Cardiol 2017;70(6):776–803.

21. Maron MS, Chan RH, Kapur NK, et al. Effect of spironolactone on myocardial fibrosis and other clinical variables in patients with hypertrophic cardiomyopathy. Am J Med 2018;131(7):837–41.

22. Elliott PM, Anastasakis A, Borger MA, et al. 2014 ESC guidelines on diagnosis and management of hypertrophic cardiomyopathy: the task force for the diagnosis and management of hypertrophic cardiomyopathy of the European Society of Cardiology (ESC). Eur Heart J 2014;35(39):2733–79.

23. Abraham WT, Fisher WG, Smith AL, et al. Cardiac resynchronization in chronic heart failure. N Engl J Med 2002;346(24):1845–53.

24. Cleland JG, Daubert JC, Erdmann E, et al. The effect of cardiac resynchronization on morbidity and mortality in heart failure. N Engl J Med 2005;352(15):1539–49.

25. D'Andrea A, Caso P, Severino S, et al. Prognostic value of intra-left ventricular electromechanical asynchrony in patients with hypertrophic cardiomyopathy. Eur Heart J 2006;27(11):1311–8.

26. Rogers DP, Marazia S, Chow AW, et al. Effect of biventricular pacing on symptoms and cardiac remodelling in patients with end-stage hypertrophic cardiomyopathy. Eur J Heart Fail 2008;10(5):507–13.

27. Siontis KC, Geske JB, Ong K, et al. Atrial fibrillation in hypertrophic cardiomyopathy: prevalence, clinical correlations, and mortality in a large high-risk population. J Am Heart Assoc 2014;3(3):e001002.

28. Saygili E, Rana OR, Saygili E, et al. Losartan prevents stretch-induced electrical remodeling in cultured atrial neonatal myocytes. Am J Physiol Heart Circ Physiol 2007;292(6):H2898–905.

29. Khatib R, Joseph P, Briel M, et al. Blockade of the renin-angiotensin-aldosterone system (RAAS) for primary prevention of non-valvular atrial fibrillation: a systematic review and meta analysis of randomized controlled trials. Int J Cardiol 2013;165(1):17–24.

30. Huang CY, Yang YH, Lin LY, et al. Renin-angiotensin-aldosterone blockade reduces atrial fibrillation in hypertrophic cardiomyopathy. Heart 2018;104(15):1276–83.

31. Patel SR, Saeed O, Naftel D, et al. Outcomes of restrictive and hypertrophic cardiomyopathies after LVAD: an INTERMACS analysis. J Card Fail 2017;23(12):859–67.

32. Topilsky Y, Pereira NL, Shah DK, et al. Left ventricular assist device therapy in patients with restrictive and hypertrophic cardiomyopathy. Circ Heart Fail 2011;4(3):266–75.

33. Maeda K, Nasirov T, Rosenthal DN, et al. An alternative approach by HVAD(R) ventricular assist device in hypertrophic cardiomyopathy. Ann Thorac Surg 2018. https://doi.org/10.1016/j.athoracsur.2018.04.065.

34. Sridharan L, Wayda B, Truby LK, et al. Mechanical circulatory support device utilization and heart transplant waitlist outcomes in patients with restrictive and hypertrophic cardiomyopathy. Circ Heart Fail 2018;11(3):e004665.

35. Zuniga Cisneros J, Stehlik J, Selzman CH, et al. Outcomes in patients with hypertrophic cardiomyopathy awaiting heart transplantation. Circ Heart Fail 2018;11(3):e004378.

36. Hsich EM, Rogers JG, McNamara DM, et al. Does survival on the heart transplant waiting list depend on the underlying heart disease? JACC Heart Fail 2016;4(9):689–97.

37. Maron MS, Kalsmith BM, Udelson JE, et al. Survival after cardiac transplantation in patients with hypertrophic cardiomyopathy. Circ Heart Fail 2010;3(5):574–9.

38. Lee MS, Zimmer R, Kobashigawa J. Long-term outcomes of orthotopic heart transplantation for hypertrophic cardiomyopathy. Transplant Proc 2014;46(5):1502–5.

Novel Pharmacotherapy for Hypertrophic Cardiomyopathy

Timothy C. Wong, MD, MS[a],*, Matthew Martinez, MD[b]

KEYWORDS

- Hypertrophic cardiomyopathy • Medical therapy • Clinical trials • Novel drug development

KEY POINTS

- Guideline recommended medical therapy for hypertrophic cardiomyopathy (HCM) remains palliative in nature.
- Off-label indications of clinically available medications are under study for HCM applications, yet none have demonstrated disease modulation ability in human studies.
- Novel medications specifically targeting HCM are under development, and preliminary data in humans warrant larger-scale study.

INTRODUCTION

Pharmacologic therapy for hypertrophic cardiomyopathy (HCM) has focused on palliation of symptoms of angina and heart failure due to left ventricular outflow tract obstruction (LVOTO) as well as diastolic dysfunction.[1] Yet, substantial treatment gaps remain in the currently available portfolio. For example, anti-inotropic medications for reduction of left ventricular outflow gradient are not always effective at control of obstruction and associated symptoms. Therapy for diastolic dysfunction in nonobstructive HCM is most effective for the subgroup who develop heart failure symptoms.[2] Furthermore, no medication has demonstrated the potential to modulate or reverse underlying disease processes, including progression of hypertrophy or diastolic dysfunction in humans.[3] In this article, a brief discussion of currently available therapy serves as a starting point to a review of both clinically available medications with novel applications for HCM and novel medications with a specific indication for HCM. Finally, a brief summary of the current gaps and potential targets for pharmacotherapy is discussed.

CURRENT GUIDELINE-RECOMMENDED MEDICAL THERAPY

The main goal of pharmacotherapy is to treat symptoms due to HCM. In patients with *obstructive* HCM, both beta-blockade and non-dihydropyridine calcium-channel blockade have been reported to decrease the LVOT gradient and improve symptoms, especially on exertion. Of note, the observation that beta and calcium-channel blockers for prevention of disease progression in asymptomatic patients has not been well established is specifically mentioned in the US guidelines.[1] Disopyramide is a useful second-line therapy with a more potent anti-inotropic effect, and its efficacy is supported by a multicenter observational trial.[4] In patients with *nonobstructive* HCM with heart failure symptoms, the overall approach is to lengthen diastolic filling time with beta-blockers or nondihydropyridine calcium-channel blockers as well as reduce left

---

[a] Department of Medicine, Division of Cardiology, University of Pittsburgh School of Medicine, UPMC Hypertrophic Cardiomyopathy Center, UPMC Heart and Vascular Institute, 200 Lothrop Street, Pittsburgh, PA 15213, USA; [b] Division of Cardiology, Lehigh Valley Health Network, 1250 South Cedar Crest Boulevard, Suite 300, Allentown, PA 18103, USA
* Corresponding author.
E-mail address: wongtc@upmc.edu

Cardiol Clin 37 (2019) 113–117
https://doi.org/10.1016/j.ccl.2018.08.008
0733-8651/19/© 2018 Elsevier Inc. All rights reserved.

ventricular (LV) diastolic filling pressures with judicious use of diuretics. Should the LV systolic function be reduced, it is assumed that the benefit of renin-angiotensin-aldosterone inhibition observed in patients with systolic heart failure apply to patients with HCM with low ejection fraction as well.[5] A discussion of the pharmacotherapy of atrial fibrillation and other arrhythmias in HCM is beyond the scope of this article, although the overall theme of palliation (as opposed to cure) remains applicable.

POTENTIAL APPLICATIONS OF CLINICALLY AVAILABLE MEDICATIONS FOR DISEASE MODULATION IN HYPERTROPHIC CARDIOMYOPATHY

Several medications already approved for other indications have demonstrated the ability to modulate disease phenotype and/or the natural progression of disease in HCM animal models. Corresponding studies in humans have for the most part not demonstrated such strong findings, although most of these studies were small and exploratory in nature and some remain ongoing. Compounds for which ample preclinical and clinical data have been published are reviewed later, and agents with more limited data are listed.

N-Acetylcysteine

N-acetylcysteine (NAC) is a precursor of glutathione, which is a potent inhibitor of oxidative stress pathways. Given associations between oxidative stress signaling pathways, myocardial metabolism, myofilament proteins, and the development of cardiac hypertrophy, it has been considered a drug of interest for potentially attenuating hypertrophy phenotypes.[6] In a mouse model of HCM, treatment with NAC reversed diastolic dysfunction and myocardial hypertrophy via oxidative myofilament modifications.[7] A feasibility study entitled Hypertrophy Regression with N-Acetylcysteine in Hypertrophic Cardiomyopathy (HALT-HCM) in which human participants with HCM were randomized to NAC versus placebo did not demonstrate large effect sizes regarding indices of hypertrophy, fibrosis, mass, and strain or functional capacity (acknowledging that the pilot study was simply not powered to identify small differences between the study groups).[6]

Renin-Angiotensin-Aldosterone System Blockade

Given the association between renin-angiotensin-aldosterone system (RAAS) regulation and a wide range of cardiovascular derangements, including vascular dysfunction, myocardial fibrosis, and cardiac hypertrophy (all phenotypes common in HCM), inhibition of fundamental pathways within the system may represent therapeutic targets of interest.[8] Further supporting this hypothesis is the observation that prohypertrophy RAAS gene polymorphisms are associated with LV hypertrophy LVH and LVOTO in human subjects with HCM.[9]

- Enalaprilat and captopril are angiotensin-converting enzyme inhibitors. A small study in human patients with HCM demonstrated improved diastolic function and coronary blood flow following intracoronary injection of enalaprilat and sublingual captopril.[10]
- Losartan, valsartan, and candesartan are angiotensin receptor blockers. In a mouse model of human HCM, losartan reversed interstitial fibrosis (and expression of collagen and transforming growth factor beta) in the heart. In humans, 4 small trials enrolling patients with nonobstructive HCM suggested improved LV function and delay of hypertrophy progression.[11–14]
- Spironolactone is an aldosterone antagonist, and its administration normalizes fibrosis levels in mouse HCM models.[15] However, a clinical trial in human HCM participants found no difference in cardiac imaging measures of cardiac remodeling over a 1-year period on spironolactone therapy.[16] An upcoming trial with a larger cohort and longer observation period may provide further insight into the impact of spironolactone on the human HCM phenotype (NCT02948998).

Diltiazem

Diltiazem is a non-dihydropyridine calcium-channel blocker that prevented the development of the HCM phenotype in a mouse model of HCM. The putative mechanism invokes sarcomeric protein mutations leading to dysregulation of intracellular calcium handling and subsequent myocyte derangement, which was not observed with the administration of L-type calcium-channel inhibitor.[17] A small randomized human pilot trial in patients with genotype positive/phenotype negative HCM with confirmed myosin binding protein-3 mutations demonstrated modest improvement in cardiac dimensions as well as serum troponin I levels in the diltiazem arm compared with the control.[18]

3-Hydroxy-3-Methylglutaryl–Coenzyme A Reductase Inhibitors (Statins)

In initial studies in a rabbit model of HCM, simvastatin led to regression of hypertrophy and myocardial fibrosis[19] and *atorvastatin* prevented the development of LVH in susceptible animals. However, small pilot studies in humans have not demonstrated detectable changes in cardiac mass or function.[20,21]

Perhexiline

Perhexiline is a coronary vasodilating agent as well as potent inhibitor of carnitine palmitoyltransferase-1 and -2, leading to increased myocardial oxygen utilization efficiency. A randomized trial of perhexiline added on to standard medical therapy demonstrated improved peak oxygen consumption (Vo_2) compared with the control.[22] Of note, the study measured phosphocreatine to adenosine triphosphate ratios in both study arms, supporting the hypothesis that perhexiline improved myocardial energetic status in hypertrophied myocardium. However, significant side effects and toxicity have been observed with its use.

Ranolazine

Ranolazine is an antianginal medication that inhibits the late sodium ion (Na^+) current in myocytes. In vitro studies using human tissue from myectomy surgery pointed to enhanced late Na^+ current contributing to abnormal intracellular calcium ion (Ca^{2+}) handling, suggesting that inhibition of the channel might serve as a therapeutic target.[23] In transgenic HCM mice, ranolazine prevented the development of the hypertrophy phenotype.[24] A small study in human patients with HCM demonstrated improvement in symptoms and quality of life in response to ranolazine.[25] However, a larger pilot study failed to demonstrate a benefit on functional capacity (peak Vo_2 measurement) or quality of life. Nonetheless, these observations regarding ranolazine served to stimulate interest in a novel, more specific inhibitor of the late Na^+ current, which is discussed in the novel medication section.

Other Medications

Propafenone, a class 1C antiarrhythmic agent with beta-blocking properties, was demonstrated to reduce LVOTO in response to IV infusion during cardiac catheterization in 11 patients with HCM.[26] *Midodrine* is a sympathomimetic agent that leads to vasoconstriction via peripheral alpha-adrenergic receptors. A case series reports improvement in LVOTO and symptoms with therapy,[27] and a clinical trial has been proposed. *Pirfenidone* is an antifibrotic agent that inhibits the transformation of fibroblasts into myofibroblasts as well as decreases the expression of known myocardial fibrosis mediators, such as transforming growth factor beta 1 and matrix metalloproteinase 9.[28,29] A clinical trial in humans has been completed, but results have not been released (NCT00011076). *Trimetazidine* is an antianginal medication that improves myocardial glucose utilization by inhibiting fatty-acid metabolism. Preliminary observations in a hamster model of HCM normalized intracellular calcium, reversed myocardial hypertrophy, and improved survival.[30] Results of initial studies in humans have not been published (NCT01696370).

NOVEL MEDICATIONS SPECIFICALLY TARGETING HYPERTROPHIC CARDIOMYOPATHY

Eleclazine

Eleclazine (GS-6615) is a novel, selective inhibitor of the late Na^+ current and is more potent and selectively inhibiting compared with ranolazine.[31] Preliminary studies were encouraging, demonstrating anti-ischemic and antiarrhythmic properties in animal models.[32] A phase 2 study was initiated in patients with HCM (LIBERTY-HCM) but terminated early following results from a parallel study in non-HCM patients showing no benefit in patients for suppression of ventricular arrhythmias (www.gilead.com).

Mavacamten

Mavacamten (MYK-461) is a small molecule that modulates cardiac myosin ATPase and directly targets the underlying sarcomere hypercontractility of HCM. The binding region where the molecule interacts with myosin corresponds to the general location on the protein structure where many pathogenic mutations of myosin heavy chain occur.[33] In mouse studies, early treatment of phenotype-negative HCM mice prevented development of hypertrophy and other hallmarks of HCM; administration to mice with the HCM phenotype attenuated hypertrophic and profibrotic gene expression as well.[34] In the initial phase 2 study of mavacamten in human patients with HCM, LVOTO gradients were significantly reduced and symptoms and functional capacity also improved.[35] The adverse effect profile was mild to moderate with most events deemed unrelated to the study drug. A phase 3 study is underway among patients with HCM with LVOTO (EXPLORER-HCM, NCT03470545), and a phase 2 study is also underway targeting nonobstructive HCM (MAVERICK-HCM, NCT03442764).

SUMMARY: CURRENT STATE OF AFFAIRS AND FUTURE DIRECTIONS

In summary, a variety of clinically available medications are in current use for the treatment of obstructive and nonobstructive HCM. Not all patients benefit from current therapy, and some progress to more advanced disease states of severe heart failure and other complications. Beyond guideline-recommended medications (beta-blockers, calcium-channel blockers, disopyramide) for symptomatic patients, several other medications have been studied with mixed results. Some have shown promise for disease palliation as well as for disease modulation in preclinical animal studies but have not panned out in initial human studies. In addition, head-to-head trials of comparative efficacy and effectiveness among the various medical therapy options are lacking. However, research efforts continue in the HCM arena with a focus on developing therapy that directly targets underlying disease processes, such as hypertrophy, fibrosis, arrhythmia, and hypercontractile states. Results of current trials involving mavacamten will be of significant interest to physicians and patients alike. Finally, gene therapy may offer an alternative approach to targeting fundamental disease processes by potentially eliminating the causative mutation for HCM itself. Although beyond the scope of this article focused on pharmacotherapy, the report of successful correction of a heterozygous MYBPC3 mutation in human embryos using a CRISPR-Cas9–based technique has raised the possibility of a cure for HCM.[36] Ultimately, time and rigorous research will inform the community of whether we are nearing the goal of targeting the fundamental pathogenesis of HCM or whether these advances join prior candidates that seemed promising in animal studies but not applicable to human use.

REFERENCES

1. Gersh BJ, Maron BJ, Bonow RO, et al. 2011 ACCF/AHA guideline for the diagnosis and treatment of hypertrophic cardiomyopathy: a report of the American College of cardiology foundation/American heart association task force on practice guidelines. Circulation 2011;124(24). https://doi.org/10.1161/CIR.0b013e318223e2bd.

2. Maron MS, Rowin EJ, Olivotto I, et al. Contemporary natural history and management of nonobstructive hypertrophic cardiomyopathy. J Am Coll Cardiol 2016;67(12):1399–409.

3. Force T, Bonow RO, Houser SR, et al. Research priorities in hypertrophic cardiomyopathy: report of a working group of the National Heart, lung, and blood institute. Circulation 2010;122(11):1130–3.

4. Sherrid MV, Barac I, Mckenna WJ, et al. Multicenter study of the efficacy and safety of disopyramide in obstructive hypertrophic cardiomyopathy. J Am Coll Cardiol 2005;45(8). https://doi.org/10.1016/j.jacc.2005.01.012.

5. Elliott PM, Anastasakis A, Borger MA, et al. 2014 ESC guidelines on diagnosis and management of hypertrophic cardiomyopathy: the task force for the diagnosis and management of hypertrophic cardiomyopathy of the European Society of Cardiology (ESC). Eur Heart J 2014;35(39):2733–79.

6. Marian AJ, Tan Y, Li L, et al. Hypertrophy regression with n-acetylcysteine in hypertrophic cardiomyopathy (HALT-HCM)novelty and significance. Circ Res 2018;122(8):1109–18.

7. Wilder T, Ryba DM, Wieczorek DF, et al. N-acetylcysteine reverses diastolic dysfunction and hypertrophy in familial hypertrophic cardiomyopathy. Am J Physiol Heart Circ Physiol 2015;309(10):H1720–30.

8. Lim HS, MacFadyen RJ, Lip GY. Diabetes mellitus, the renin-angiotensin-aldosterone system, and the heart. Arch Intern Med 2004;164(16):1737–48.

9. Kaufman BD, Auerbach S, Reddy S, et al. RAAS gene polymorphisms influence progression of pediatric hypertrophic cardiomyopathy. Hum Genet 2007;122(5):515–23.

10. Kyriakidis M, Triposkiadis F, Dernellis J, et al. Effects of cardiac versus circulatory angiotensin-converting enzyme inhibition on left ventricular diastolic function and coronary blood flow in hypertrophic obstructive cardiomyopathy. Circulation 1998;97(14):1342–7.

11. Kawano H, Toda G, Nakamizo R, et al. Valsartan decreases type I collagen synthesis in patients with hypertrophic cardiomyopathy. Circ J 2005;69(10):1244–8. Available at: http://www.ncbi.nlm.nih.gov/pubmed/16195625. Accessed August 6, 2018.

12. Yamazaki T, Suzuki J-I, Shimamoto R, et al. A new therapeutic strategy for hypertrophic nonobstructive cardiomyopathy in humans. A randomized and prospective study with an Angiotensin II receptor blocker. Int Heart J 2007;48(6):715–24. Available at: http://www.ncbi.nlm.nih.gov/pubmed/18160763. Accessed August 6, 2018.

13. Penicka M, Gregor P, Kerekes R, et al. The effects of candesartan on left ventricular hypertrophy and function in nonobstructive hypertrophic cardiomyopathy. J Mol Diagn 2009;11(1):35–41.

14. Araujo AQ, Arteaga E, Ianni BM, et al. Effect of Losartan on left ventricular diastolic function in patients with nonobstructive hypertrophic cardiomyopathy. Am J Cardiol 2005;96(11):1563–7.

15. Tsybouleva N, Zhang L, Chen S, et al. Aldosterone, through novel signaling proteins, is a fundamental molecular bridge between the genetic defect and the cardiac phenotype of hypertrophic cardiomyopathy. Circulation 2004;109(10):1284–91.

16. Maron MS, Chan RH, Kapur NK, et al. Effect of spironolactone on myocardial fibrosis and other clinical

variables in patients with hypertrophic cardiomyopathy. Am J Med 2018;131(7):837–41.

17. Semsarian C, Ahmad I, Giewat M, et al. The L-type calcium channel inhibitor diltiazem prevents cardiomyopathy in a mouse model. J Clin Invest 2002; 109(8):1013–20.

18. Ho CY, Lakdawala NK, Cirino AL, et al. Diltiazem treatment for pre-Clinical hypertrophic cardiomyopathy sarcomere Mutation carriers: a pilot randomized trial to modify disease expression. JACC Heart Fail 2015;3(2):180–8.

19. Patel R, Nagueh SF, Tsybouleva N, et al. Simvastatin induces regression of cardiac hypertrophy and fibrosis and improves cardiac function in a transgenic rabbit model of human hypertrophic cardiomyopathy. Circulation 2001;104(3):317–24.

20. Nagueh SF, Lombardi R, Tan Y, et al. Atorvastatin and cardiac hypertrophy and function in hypertrophic cardiomyopathy: a pilot study. Eur J Clin Invest 2010;40(11):976–83.

21. Hersi A, Giannoccaro JP, Howarth A, et al. Statin induced regression of cardiomyopathy trial: a randomized, placebo-controlled double-blind trial. Heart Views 2016;17(4):129–35.

22. Abozguia K, Elliott P, McKenna W, et al. Metabolic modulator perhexiline corrects energy deficiency and improves exercise capacity in symptomatic hypertrophic cardiomyopathy. Circulation 2010; 122(16):1562–9.

23. Coppini R, Ferrantini C, Yao L, et al. Late sodium current inhibition reverses electromechanical dysfunction in human hypertrophic cardiomyopathy. Circulation 2013;127(5):575–84.

24. Coppini R, Mazzoni L, Ferrantini C, et al. Ranolazine prevents phenotype development in a mouse model of hypertrophic cardiomyopathy. Circ Heart Fail 2017;10(3):1–17.

25. Gentry JL, Mentz RJ, Hurdle M, et al. Ranolazine for treatment of angina or dyspnea in hypertrophic cardiomyopathy patients (RHYME). J Am Coll Cardiol 2016;68(16):1815–7.

26. Funck F, Bourmayan C, Cristofini P, et al. Hemodynamic effects on intravenous propafenone in hypertrophic myocardiopathy. Arch Mal Coeur Vaiss 1988;81(4):525–9 [in French]. Available at: http://www.ncbi.nlm.nih.gov/pubmed/3136714. Accessed August 6, 2018.

27. Lafitte S, Peyrou J, Reynaud A, et al. Midodrine hydrochloride and unexpected improvement in hypertrophic cardiomyopathy symptoms. Arch Cardiovasc Dis 2016;109(3):223–5.

28. Shi Q, Liu X, Bai Y, et al. In vitro effects of pirfenidone on cardiac fibroblasts: proliferation, myofibroblast differentiation, migration and cytokine secretion. PLoS One 2011;6(11):e28134.

29. Tamargo J, López-Sendón J. Novel therapeutic targets for the treatment of heart failure. Nat Rev Drug Discov 2011;10(7):536–55.

30. D'hahan N, Taouil K, Janmot C, et al. Effect of trimetazidine and verapamil on the cardiomyopathic hamster myosin phenotype. Br J Pharmacol 1998; 123(4):611–6.

31. Olivotto I, Hellawell JL, Farzaneh-Far R, et al. Novel approach targeting the complex pathophysiology of hypertrophic cardiomyopathy: the impact of late sodium current inhibition on exercise capacity in subjects with symptomatic hypertrophic cardiomyopathy (LIBERTY-HCM) trial. Circ Hear Fail 2016;9(3):1–11.

32. Zablocki JA, Elzein E, Li X, et al. Discovery of dihydrobenzoxazepinone (GS-6615) late sodium current inhibitor (late I_{Na} i), a phase II agent with demonstrated preclinical anti-ischemic and antiarrhythmic properties. J Med Chem 2016;59(19):9005–17.

33. Kawas RF, Anderson RL, Ingle SRB, et al. A small-molecule modulator of cardiac myosin acts on multiple stages of the myosin chemomechanical cycle. J Biol Chem 2017;292(40):16571–7.

34. Green EM, Wakimoto H, Anderson RL, et al. Heart disease: a small-molecule inhibitor of sarcomere contractility suppresses hypertrophic cardiomyopathy in mice. Science 2016;351(6273):617–21.

35. MyoKardia Press Release. Press release. 2018. Available at: http://investors.myokardia.com/phoenix.zhtml?c=254211&p=irol-newsArticle&ID=2337154%0AWC%0A. Accessed June 8, 2018.

36. Ma H, Marti-Gutierrez N, Park S-W, et al. Correction of a pathogenic gene mutation in human embryos. Nature 2017;548(7668):413–9.

Printed and bound by CPI Group (UK) Ltd, Croydon, CR0 4YY

03/10/2024

01040385-0009